PREGNANCY AND BIRTH OUTCOMES

Edited by **Wei Wu**

Pregnancy and Birth Outcomes
http://dx.doi.org/10.5772/intechopen.69365
Edited by Wei Wu

Contributors

Qiuqin Tang, Jing Yang, Qing Xia, Andrey Momot, Maria Nikolaeva, Valeriy Elykomov, Ksenia Momot, Georg Schmolzer, Gianluca Lista, Ilia Bresesti, Yasmin H Neggers, Wei Wu

First published in London, United Kingdom, 2018 by IntechOpen
IntechOpen is the global imprint of INTECHOPEN LIMITED, registered in England and Wales, registration number: 11086078, The Shard, 25th floor, 32 London Bridge Street
London, SE19SG – United Kingdom
Printed in Croatia

British Library Cataloguing-in-Publication Data
A catalogue record for this book is available from the British Library

Additional hard copies can be obtained from orders@intechopen.com

Pregnancy and Birth Outcomes, Edited by Wei Wu
p. cm.
Print ISBN 978-1-78923-242-4
Online ISBN 978-1-78923-243-1

For EU product safety concerns:
IN TECH d.o.o., Prolaz Marije Krucifikse Kozulić 3, 51000 Rijeka, Croatia,
info@intechopen.com or visit our website at intechopen.com.

Meet the editor

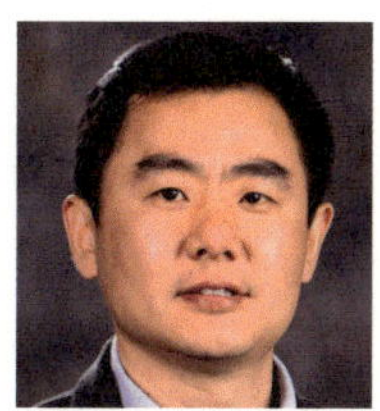

Dr. Wei Wu is an associate professor in the Institute of Toxicology, School of Public Health at Nanjing Medical University, China. He received his PhD degree in Toxicology from Nanjing Medical University in 2012. Since 2017, he is a guest researcher at NIEHS. He is a member of different national and international societies in human reproduction and toxicology field. He has been awarded by many national societies for originality and the quality of his projects. He has a wide range of teaching and consulting experiences including toxicology. His areas of expertise and interests are toxicology, male infertility, pregnancy complications, fetal growth, epigenetics, endocrine-disrupting chemicals, transgenerational effect, and reproduction and development. He has published 62 papers in international journals such as Environment International, Scientific Reports, Human Reproduction, Human Molecular Genetics, and Toxicological Sciences. He has collaborated in five books and eleven patents and in the organization of two international conferences. He is an associate editor of the *JSM Invitro Fertilization*, executive editor of *Annals of Molecular and Genetic Medicine*, and editor of *Scientific Reports, Austin Journal of Reproductive Medicine & Infertility*, and many more journals.

Contents

Preface

Despite recent advances in obstetric medicine, pregnancy complications and adverse birth outcomes are a growing public health concern and economic burden on the healthcare system. More than 10% of the global burden of disease is due to pregnancy complications and adverse birth outcomes. This book will focus on pregnancy complications and birth outcomes, from the aspects of gestational age; environmental, genetic, epigenetic risk factors, and delivery room management.

Chapter 1 is the introductory chapter. The chapter outlines environmental, genetic, and epigenetic risk factors of pregnancy complications and adverse birth outcomes. The chapter ends with an emphasis on epigenetic changes that modulate the long-term and transgenerational health effects of prenatal environmental exposure.

Chapter 2 covers the association between gestational age and some significant pregnancy outcomes, such as preterm birth, low birth weight, stillbirth, fetal growth restriction, and certain chronic diseases. This chapter also discusses race and ethnicity and low birth weight.

Chapter 3 discusses on the perinatal effects and long-term influences of maternal smoking and passive smoking during pregnancy. The first half of the chapter discusses the perinatal and neonatal effects of maternal cigarette smoking during pregnancy. The second half discusses the effects of passive smoking, the epigenetic mechanism of adverse effect of smoking during pregnancy, and antismoking measures.

Chapter 4 presents the results of association between FVL and the development of venous thromboembolic complications and gestational complications such as preeclampsia, fetal growth restriction, and miscarriage in the prospective cohort of 500 females during 2008–2015. The found patterns can be useful in assessing the need for heparin prophylaxis for FVL patients during pregnancy from the standpoint of personalized medicine.

Chapter 5 overviews the most relevant measures to manage respiratory distress syndrome from the delivery room, starting from an explanation of the disease and moving toward the most recent evidence, from the basic concepts to the most advanced techniques to monitor fetal neonatal transition.

There are many individuals who made this book a reality. The completion of this book would not have been possible without the efforts of numerous contributors. I would like to thank Mr. Teo Kos of IntechOpen for his strong support from the inception to completion of this book. I would also like to acknowledge my coauthors for their efforts.

Wei Wu
Institute of Toxicology
School of Public Health
Nanjing Medical University, China

Chapter 1

Introductory Chapter: Environmental, Genetic, and Epigenetic Risk Factors in Adverse Pregnancy and Birth Outcomes

Wei Wu

Additional information is available at the end of the chapter

http://dx.doi.org/10.5772/intechopen.76902

1. Introduction

It is well established that pregnancy complications and adverse birth outcomes are important public health concerns in both developed and developing countries. Prenatal development refers to the process in which an embryo and later fetus develop during gestation. Each pregnancy can be divided into three trimesters of approximately 3 months each. A normal, full-term pregnancy lasts about 40 weeks. During the 40 weeks of pregnancy, the embryo and fetus are heavily influenced by environment (**Figure 1**).

The human placenta is the highly specialized organ of pregnancy that is responsible normal fetal growth and development [1]. It plays an important role in substance exchange between the

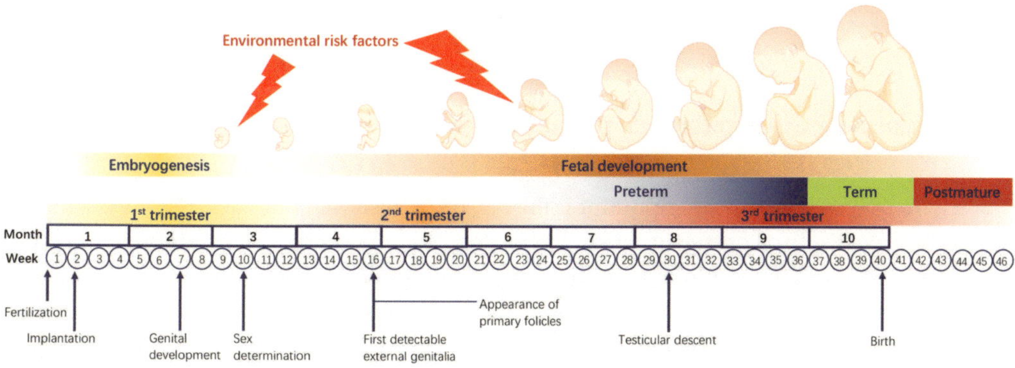

Figure 1. The embryo and fetus are heavily influenced by environment during the 40 weeks of pregnancy.

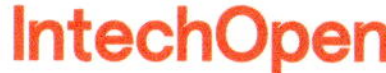

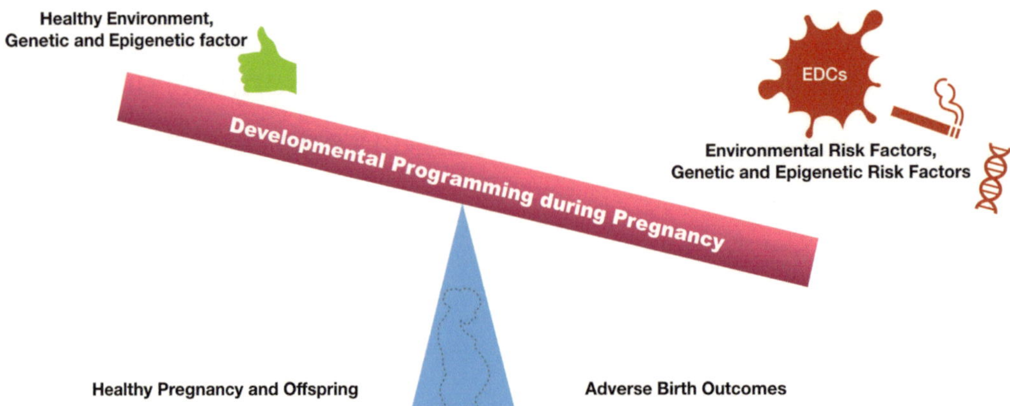

Figure 2. Several risk factors may affect fetal growth and development during pregnancy.

mother and the fetus during pregnancy. Many chemicals can transfer across the placenta and influence the development of the embryo and fetus [2]. The fetus is unable to detoxify substances efficiently because of their weak capability to detoxify toxic chemicals. Additionally, there are many different factors which can cause abnormalities of the placenta, such as environmental risk factors [3], genetic risk factors [4], and epigenetic risk factors [5]. Several studies have demonstrated that placental disorders are associated with pregnancy complications and adverse birth outcomes, including gestational diabetes mellitus (GDM), preeclampsia, miscarriage, preterm birth, stillbirth, macrosomia, and fetal growth restriction (FGR) [6–9]. The cause of pregnancy complications and adverse birth outcomes remains largely unknown but accumulating evidence have proved that environmental risk factors, genetic risk factors, and epigenetic risk factors may play important roles in the etiology and susceptibility of these diseases (**Figure 2**).

The pathogenesis of adverse pregnancy and birth outcomes is multifactorial, involving complex interactions between environmental influences, genetics, and epigenetic mechanisms. This introductory chapter mainly discusses the evidence linking several kinds of risk factors and adverse pregnancy and birth outcomes, such as environmental risk factors, genetic risk factors, and epigenetic risk factors.

2. Environmental impacts on prenatal development

The environment can have an important influence on fetal development. Variety of chemicals have been reported to be present in urine, blood, and amniotic fluid, which indicated that pregnant women around the world are highly exposed to chemicals [10–12]. Additionally, several studies also have shown that a wide range of chemicals has been detected in cord blood and fetal tissues, including bisphenol-A (BPA), phthalates, pesticides, and heavy metals [10, 13].

Environmental risk factors have a deleterious effect on prenatal development leading to problems including premature birth, stillbirth, and low birth weight [14–16]. While environmental hazards pose a definite threat to the developing fetus, they do not always cause adverse effects. The harmful health effect of environmental risk factors is determined by the timing of the exposure, the dose/duration of the exposure, genetic susceptibility, and gene-environment interactions [17, 18]. The fetus is particularly vulnerable to environmental hazards that disrupt developmental processes during relatively narrow developmental periods. For example, a birth cohort study of 1390 women found that arsenic concentrations in the third trimester, but not in the first and second trimesters, were negatively associated with birth weight and birth length [19]. Therefore, the timing of exposure during pregnancy is an important factor that may influence the outcome of exposure.

Multiple environmental risk factors, such as exposure to endocrine disrupting chemicals (EDCs), smoking, air pollution, can have a range of impacts on the health of a growing fetus [20, 21]. EDCs have the potential to interfere with endogenous hormone action. Several studies have suggested adverse endocrine disruptive effects of EDCs on the fetus, such as miscarriage, low birth weight, hypospadias, cryptorchidism, and other birth defects [20, 22]. For example, BPA is an EDC that is ubiquitous in modern environments, which provides great potential for exposure of the developing fetus. Links between BPA and endocrine disruption has been implicated in the etiology of several kinds of adverse reproductive outcomes [23, 24]. There is a large body of evidence showing that maternal smoking during pregnancy and secondhand smoking exposure can result in placental problems (previa and/or abruption), miscarriage, stillbirth, premature birth, and FGR [25, 26]. However, quitting smoking (even during pregnancy) greatly reduces the risks of these problems [25].

Although a large number of studies have examined the association between environmental risk factors exposure during pregnancy and adverse pregnancy and birth outcomes, the molecular mechanism of environment-induced adverse pregnancy and birth outcomes is still not fully understood. Thus, further researches are needed to investigate the molecular mechanisms underlying environment-induced adverse pregnancy and birth outcomes.

3. Genetic risk factors and pregnancy complications and adverse birth outcomes

It has been estimated that single nucleotide polymorphisms constitute approximately 90% of all genetic variations in the human populations. Over the past few decades, a number of epidemiologic studies, using both the candidate gene and genome-wide approach, have examined associations between genetic variants and the risk of pregnancy complications and adverse birth outcomes, such as GDM, preeclampsia, preterm birth, small for gestational age, and birth defects [18, 27–30]. Several genetic loci in genes have been identified to be associated with risks of pregnancy complications and adverse birth outcomes [27–29].

Several studies have found that gene polymorphism plays important roles in the susceptibility of pregnancy complications and adverse birth outcomes. A study conducted in the SCOPE pregnancy cohort found that the maternal and infant *FTO* (rs9939609) polymorphism AA genotype was significantly associated with increased risk of small for gestational age pregnancy and spontaneous preterm birth [31]. In a meta-analysis, Zhang et al. identified that nine polymorphisms in seven genes involved in the regulation of insulin secretion were significantly associated with risk of GDM. Among the nine polymorphisms, the rs7903146 in

TCF7L2 showed the strongest association with risk of GDM [27]. The *MTHFR* C677T polymorphism as a common genetic cause for hyperhomocysteinemia was associated with hypertension in pregnancy, preterm birth, and low birth weight [32, 33]. Nurk et al. examined the association between two polymorphisms of *MTHFR* gene (677C > T and 1298A > C) and pregnancy complications, adverse outcomes, and birth defects in 5883 women of the Hordaland Homocysteine Study. They found that the maternal carriage of the *MTHFR* 677C > T polymorphism was associated with the risk of placental abruption. However, they did not find significant associations between *MTHFR* polymorphisms and birth defects [34].

Though a large number of epidemiologic studies have examined the association between gene polymorphisms and adverse pregnancy and birth outcomes, a large portion of the results are inconsistent. Therefore, future studies with larger sample size, genomic-wide association studies (GWAS), and large-scale replications of identified associations are needed to illustrate the most significant genetic variants that associated with risk of adverse pregnancy and birth outcomes. Furthermore, as the genetic association of a polymorphism with adverse pregnancy and birth outcomes does not equate to a casual role, functional analysis should be performed to identify the causal variants.

4. Epigenetics and adverse pregnancy and birth outcomes

In addition to the sequence of the genome, the contribution of epigenetics to adverse pregnancy and birth outcomes is increasingly recognized. Epigenetics refers to heritable changes in gene expression patterns which do not alter DNA sequence. Epigenetics is now recognized as playing an important role in the etiology of human disease [7, 35, 36]. The main epigenetic mechanisms responsible for adverse pregnancy and birth outcomes are represented by DNA methylation, histone modifications, and noncoding RNA [37].

A growing body of evidence demonstrates that aberrant epigenetic modifications are associated with adverse pregnancy and birth outcomes [9, 38]. Using 1030 placental samples, Reichetzeder and colleagues reported that global placental DNA methylation was significantly increased in women with GDM [9]. In the study by Côté et al., maternal glycemia at the second and third trimester of pregnancy is correlated with variations in DNA methylation levels at *PRDM16*, *BMP7*, and *PPARGC1α* and with cord blood leptin levels [38].

The epigenetic signature inherited from the gametes is erased and established after fertilization [39]. The requirement of a high degree of spatial-temporal coordination of epigenetic changes during this process provides opportunities for disruption by environmental chemicals [40]. Unlike inherited genetic variation that is static through the course of a lifetime, epigenetic changes are sensitive indicators of the effects of acute and chronic environmental exposure [41]. Epigenetic mechanisms have been shown to be influenced by environmental factors. Abnormal epigenetic modifications represent an important mechanism for environmental factors influencing the risk of adverse pregnancy and birth outcomes. Exposure to EDCs during pregnancy has been shown to influence epigenetic programming of endocrine signaling and other important physiological pathways, thus further disrupt normal fetal development [42, 43]. The low-dose BPA administration to pregnant mice has been found to cause hypomethylation at NotI loci that is involved in brain development [44]. Recent animal study has reported that prenatal exposure to di-n-butyl phthalate (DBP) can lead to marked changes in the epigenetic regulation of gene expression [45].

Previous studies have demonstrated that prenatal exposure to some EDCs (such as vinclozolin, methoxychlor, DBP, and DDT) may cause the transgenerational effect of adult disease [45, 46]. In recent years, a growing body of research has spotlighted the role of epigenetic mechanism in the transgenerational effect of prenatal exposure to EDCs [45–47]. Many of the environmentally induced epigenetic changes can be transmitted to future generations and associated with disease phenotypes in the unexposed individuals of subsequent generations. It has been reported that prenatal exposure to DBP may have the transgenerational effect of spermatogenic failure [45]. These adverse outcomes were accompanied by global DNA hypomethylation and spermatogenesis modulator gene (*Fstl3*) promoter hypomethylation, suggesting that prenatal DBP exposure can be imprinted through epigenetic alterations. Additionally, epigenetic markers may be useful as biomarkers for environmental exposure and disease and as potential targets for preventive and therapeutic interventions [48, 49].

This chapter puts an updated overview of the risk factors of adverse pregnancy outcomes and birth outcomes, transgenerational effect of prenatal environmental exposure on health in later life, and epigenetic mechanisms of environmental risk factor-induced adverse pregnancy outcomes and birth outcomes. By this way, these observations can be used to advise pregnant women or women of reproductive age to avoid such exposures and adopt a positive lifestyle to protect pregnancy and normal fetal development. Overall, avoidance of potential risk factors, identification of high susceptible women, and provision of personalized medical care are important in the healthcare management of pregnant women.

Author details

Wei Wu

Address all correspondence to: wwu@njmu.edu.cn

Nanjing Medical University, Nanjing, China

References

[1] John R, Hemberger M. A placenta for life. Reproductive Biomedicine Online. 2012;**25**:5-11

[2] Giaginis C, Theocharis S, Tsantili-Kakoulidou A. Current toxicological aspects on drug and chemical transport and metabolism across the human placental barrier. Expert Opinion on Drug Metabolism & Toxicology. 2012;**8**:1263-1275

[3] Vrooman LA, Xin F, Bartolomei MS. Morphologic and molecular changes in the placenta: What we can learn from environmental exposures. Fertility and Sterility. 2016; **106**:930-940

[4] Gundacker C et al. Genetics of the human placenta: Implications for toxicokinetics. Archives of Toxicology. 2016;**90**:2563-2581

[5] Vaiman D. Genes, epigenetics and miRNA regulation in the placenta. Placenta. 2017; **52**:127-133

[6] Khot VV et al. Hypermethylated CpG sites in the MTR gene promoter in preterm placenta. Epigenomics. 2017;**9**:985-996

[7] Li J et al. The role, mechanism and potentially novel biomarker of microRNA-17-92 cluster in macrosomia. Scientific Reports. 2015;**5**:17212

[8] Tang Q et al. miR-141 contributes to fetal growth restriction by regulating PLAG1 expression. PLoS One. 2013;**8**:e58737

[9] Reichetzeder C et al. Increased global placental DNA methylation levels are associated with gestational diabetes. Clinical Epigenetics. 2016;**8**:82

[10] Maekawa R et al. Evidence of exposure to chemicals and heavy metals during pregnancy in Japanese women. Reproductive Medicine and Biology. 2017;**16**:337-348

[11] Tefre de Renzy-Martin K et al. Current exposure of 200 pregnant Danish women to phthalates, parabens and phenols. Reproduction. 2014;**147**:443-453

[12] Shekhar S et al. Detection of phenolic endocrine disrupting chemicals (EDCs) from maternal blood plasma and amniotic fluid in Indian population. General and Comparative Endocrinology. 2017;**241**:100-107

[13] Gerona RR et al. Bisphenol-A (BPA), BPA glucuronide, and BPA sulfate in midgestation umbilical cord serum in a Northern and Central California population. Environmental Science & Technology. 2013;**47**:12477-12485

[14] Cantonwine DE, Ferguson KK, Mukherjee B, McElrath TF, Meeker JD. Urinary bisphenol A levels during pregnancy and risk of preterm birth. Environmental Health Perspectives. 2015;**123**:895-901

[15] Yang S et al. Ambient air pollution the risk of stillbirth: A prospective birth cohort study in Wuhan, China. International Journal of Hygiene and Environmental Health. 2018. Pii: S1438-4639(17)30531-X

[16] Smith RB et al. Impact of London's road traffic air and noise pollution on birth weight: Retrospective population based cohort study. BMJ. 2017;**359**:j5299

[17] Arroyo V, Diaz J, Carmona R, Ortiz C, Linares C. Impact of air pollution and temperature on adverse birth outcomes: Madrid, 2001-2009. Environmental Pollution. 2016;**218**:1154-1161

[18] Hong X et al. Genome-wide approach identifies a novel gene-maternal pre-pregnancy BMI interaction on preterm birth. Nature Communications. 2017;**8**:15608

[19] Liu H et al. Maternal arsenic exposure and birth outcomes: A birth cohort study in Wuhan, China. Environmental Pollution. 2018;**236**:817-823

[20] Krieg SA, Shahine LK, Lathi RB. Environmental exposure to endocrine-disrupting chemicals and miscarriage. Fertility and Sterility. 2016;**106**:941-947

[21] Polanska K et al. Environmental tobacco smoke exposure during pregnancy and child neurodevelopment. International Journal of Environmental Research and Public Health. 2017;**14**. pii: E796

[22] Zhang Y et al. Phthalate levels and low birth weight: A nested case-control study of Chinese newborns. The Journal of Pediatrics. 2009;**155**:500-504

[23] Fernandez MF et al. Bisphenol A and other phenols in human placenta from children with cryptorchidism or hypospadias. Reproductive Toxicology. 2016;**59**:89-95

[24] Barrett ES et al. First-trimester urinary bisphenol A concentration in relation to anogenital distance, an androgen-sensitive measure of reproductive development, in infant girls. Environmental Health Perspectives. 2017;**125**:077008

[25] Phelan S. Smoking cessation in pregnancy. Obstetrics and Gynecology Clinics of North America. 2014;**41**:255-266

[26] Ananth CV, Savitz DA, Luther ER. Maternal cigarette smoking as a risk factor for placental abruption, placenta previa, and uterine bleeding in pregnancy. American Journal of Epidemiology. 1996;**144**:881-889

[27] Zhang C et al. Genetic variants and the risk of gestational diabetes mellitus: A systematic review. Human Reproduction Update. 2013;**19**:376-390

[28] Stalman SE et al. Genetic analyses in small-for-gestational-age newborns. The Journal of Clinical Endocrinology and Metabolism. 2018;**103**:917-925

[29] Yong HEJ, Murthi P, Brennecke SP, Moses EK. Genetic approaches in preeclampsia. Methods in Molecular Biology. 2018;**1710**:53-72

[30] Jin SC et al. Contribution of rare inherited and de novo variants in 2871 congenital heart disease probands. Nature Genetics. 2017;**49**:1593-1601

[31] Andraweera PH et al. The obesity associated FTO gene variant and the risk of adverse pregnancy outcomes: Evidence from the SCOPE study. Obesity (Silver Spring). 2016; **24**:2600-2607

[32] Yang B et al. Associations of MTHFR gene polymorphisms with hypertension and hypertension in pregnancy: A meta-analysis from 114 studies with 15411 cases and 21970 controls. PLoS One. 2014;**9**:e87497

[33] Wu H et al. Genetic polymorphism of MTHFR C677T with preterm birth and low birth weight susceptibility: A meta-analysis. Archives of Gynecology and Obstetrics. 2017;**295**:1105-1118

[34] Nurk E, Tell GS, Refsum H, Ueland PM, Vollset SE. Associations between maternal methylenetetrahydrofolate reductase polymorphisms and adverse outcomes of

pregnancy: The Hordaland Homocysteine Study. The American Journal of Medicine. 2004;**117**:26-31

[35] Weinhold B. Epigenetics: The science of change. Environmental Health Perspectives. 2006;**114**:A160-A167

[36] Wu W et al. Genome-wide microRNA expression profiling in idiopathic non-obstructive azoospermia: Significant up-regulation of miR-141, miR-429 and miR-7-1-3p. Human Reproduction. 2013;**28**:1827-1836

[37] Nelissen EC, van Montfoort AP, Dumoulin JC, Evers JL. Epigenetics and the placenta. Human Reproduction Update. 2011;**17**:397-417

[38] Côté S et al. PPARGC1alpha gene DNA methylation variations in human placenta mediate the link between maternal hyperglycemia and leptin levels in newborns. Clinical Epigenetics. 2016;**8**:72

[39] Heard E, Martienssen RA. Transgenerational epigenetic inheritance: Myths and mechanisms. Cell. 2014;**157**:95-109

[40] Ho SM et al. Environmental factors, epigenetics, and developmental origin of reproductive disorders. Reproductive Toxicology. 2017;**68**:85-104

[41] Bommarito PA, Martin E, Fry RC. Effects of prenatal exposure to endocrine disruptors and toxic metals on the fetal epigenome. Epigenomics. 2017;**9**:333-350

[42] Fudvoye J, Bourguignon JP, Parent AS. Endocrine-disrupting chemicals and human growth and maturation: A focus on early critical windows of exposure. Vitamins and Hormones. 2014;**94**:1-25

[43] Vilahur N et al. Prenatal exposure to mixtures of xenoestrogens and repetitive element DNA methylation changes in human placenta. Environment International. 2014;**71**:81-87

[44] Yaoi T et al. Genome-wide analysis of epigenomic alterations in fetal mouse forebrain after exposure to low doses of bisphenol A. Biochemical and Biophysical Research Communications. 2008;**376**:563-567

[45] Yuan B et al. From the cover: Metabolomics reveals a role of betaine in prenatal DBP exposure-induced epigenetic transgenerational failure of spermatogenesis in rats. Toxicological Sciences. 2017;**158**:356-366

[46] Anway MD, Cupp AS, Uzumcu M, Skinner MK. Epigenetic transgenerational actions of endocrine disruptors and male fertility. Science. 2005;**308**:1466-1469

[47] Skinner MK et al. Alterations in sperm DNA methylation, non-coding RNA and histone retention associate with DDT-induced epigenetic transgenerational inheritance of disease. Epigenetics & Chromatin. 2018;**11**:8

[48] Laufer BI, Chater-Diehl EJ, Kapalanga J, Singh SM. Long-term alterations to DNA methylation as a biomarker of prenatal alcohol exposure: From mouse models to human children with fetal alcohol spectrum disorders. Alcohol. 2017;**60**:67-75

[49] Subramaniam D, Thombre R, Dhar A, Anant S. DNA methyltransferases: A novel target for prevention and therapy. Frontiers in Oncology. 2014;**4**:80

Chapter 2

Gestational Age and Pregnancy Outcomes

Yasmin H. Neggers

Additional information is available at the end of the chapter

http://dx.doi.org/10.5772/intechopen.72419

Abstract

Some of the important pregnancy outcomes such as preterm delivery, growth restriction and low birth weight (LBW) infant, stillbirth, and some long-term chronic diseases vary by race and ethnicity but also tend to be associated with gestational age of the infant at birth. In the United States, during the last 25–30 years, the rate of low birth weight has increased, as has the rate of preterm delivery among both whites and blacks. Examination of causes for these secular trends has focused mainly on changes in the distribution of maternal age, race, and certain psychosocial factors. However, gestational age at birth is associated with most of these pregnancy outcomes, particularly infant mortality, certain morbidities, birth weight, and preterm birth. In this chapter, the association between gestational age and some significant pregnancy outcomes will be discussed.

Keywords: gestational age, pregnancy outcome, infant mortality, preterm, growth restriction

1. Introduction

Before illustrating the significance of gestational age at birth and pregnancy outcomes, definitions and information about various terms to be used in the text will be provided.

Gestational age at birth: Is defined as the time between conception and birth of an infant. The most common method of measuring gestational age in weeks is by calculating the time since the last menstrual period based on datesprovided by a woman at the first prenatal visit [1]. A normal pregnancy period is usually between 38 and 40 weeks.

Appropriate for gestational age (AGA): if the infant's gestational age findings after birth match the calendar age, the infant is said to be appropriate for gestational age. The weight for full-term infants born AGA is often between 2500 and 4000 g [2].

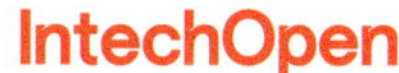

Small for gestational age (SGA): infants weighing less than 2500 g are considered small for gestational age.

Large for gestational age (SGA): infants weighing more than 4000 g are considered large for gestational age.

Low birth weight (LBW): is not a homogeneous pregnancy outcome, but, instead, is composed of infants who are either born too early, that is, preterm birth, or too small, that is, fetal growth restriction [3]. A LBW infant, according to the World Health Organization, is born weighing <2500 g [4].

Preterm birth (premature birth): is the birth of a baby at fewer than 37 weeks of gestation. Preterm birth can be spontaneous or induced [5]. **Figure 1** illustrates a combination of categories of preterm birth, low birth weight, and small for gestational age infants.

Intrauterine growth retardation (fetal growth retardation or growth restriction): growth-restricted infants or infants with intrauterine growth retardation are those born weighing less than the tenth percentile of birth weight for gestational age, regardless of whether the weight is <2500 g. Therefore, it is possible for both preterm and growth-restricted infants to weigh less than <2500. Thus to define IUGR or grow restriction, a birth weight for gestational age standard with the tenth percentile birth weight defined is needed [6, 7].

Important pregnancy outcomes include neonatal mortality, stillbirth, long-term neurologic problems, and maternal mortality [3]. Research conducted in this area indicates that many of these outcomes are associated with length of gestation or gestational age of the infant at birth. In the United States and other developed countries, pregnancy outcomes are much better than those in many developing countries, where the adverse outcomes mentioned above are increased 10–100-fold as compared to US rates [3]. However, adverse pregnancy outcomes are generally more common in the United States than other developed countries [5, 8]. Low infant birth weight, either due to preterm birth or intrauterine growth restriction, is attributed to much of the infant mortality, morbidity, and increased cost of perinatal care. Data from the US Center for Disease Control and Prevention indicates that the infant mortality rate in the United States

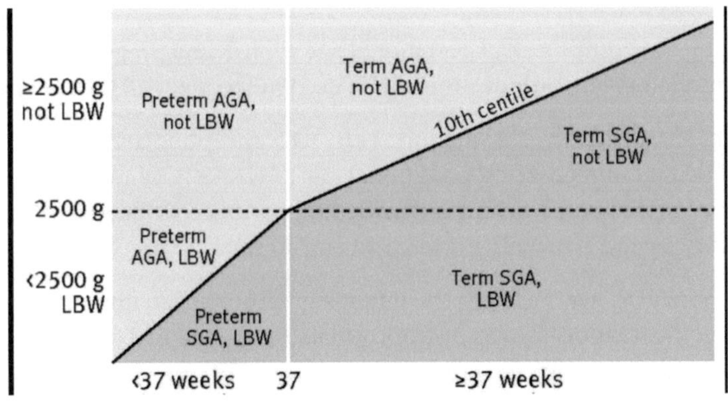

Figure 1. A combination of preterm, low birth weight, and small for gestational age infants.

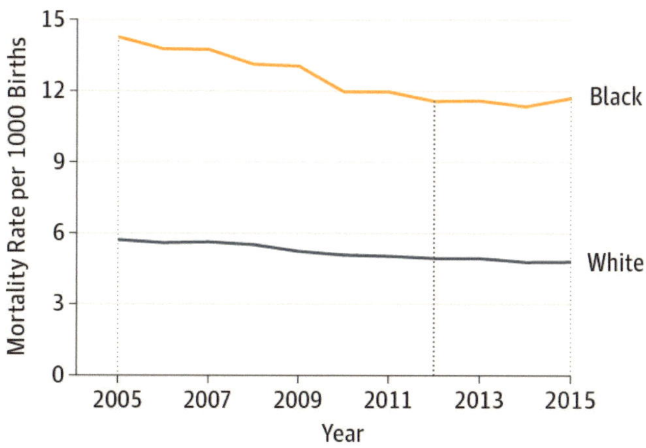

Figure 2. Infant mortality rate of black versus white infants.

during the past decade has decreased by 15% [5, 7]. Wide disparity exists in both preterm and growth restrictions among different population groups. Poor blacks, for example, have twice the preterm birth rate and higher growth restriction than do most women [5]. The infant mortality from 2005 to 2012 for non-Hispanic blacks decreased from 14.3 to 11.6/1000 births; thereafter the infant mortality rate plateaued and then increased from 11.4 to 11.7 over this time period. For non-Hispanic white infants, the rate decreased monotonically from 5.7 to 4.8/1000 births [8]. Further analyses indicate that black infants are nearly 2.2 times more likely to die than white infants during their first year of life. The trends in cause-specific mortality for four leading causes of infant death show that short gestation/low birth weight is responsible for the highest mortality rate/1000 births. Riddell et al. indicate that the gestational age at birth explains a large portion of excess deaths in black infants as compared to white infants, for example, the preterm (gestational age < 37 weeks) rate is almost 50% higher in black than to white infants [8]. Also, black infants experience nearly four times as many deaths related to short gestation and low birth weight, making it the leading cause of infant deaths among black infants during the first year of life [8]. See **Figure 2**. Thus, these results confirm that gestational age at birth is a significant factor which affects major factors resulting in poor pregnancy outcomes such as infant mortality and morbidity. The risk of adverse consequences declines with increasing gestational age [9].

In this chapter, pregnancy outcomes and its relationship to gestational age will be limited to pregnancy outcomes associated with preterm birth, race and ethnicity, low birth weight, stillbirth, small for gestational age (fetal growth restriction), and certain chronic diseases.

2. Preterm births and gestational age at birth

As noted before, preterm birth is defined as infants born before completing gestational age of 37 weeks. In 2010, an estimated 14.9 million babies were born preterm, 11.1% of all live births worldwide, ranging from about 5.5% in most European countries to 18% in some African countries [10]. Preterm birth also affects affluent countries, for example, the United States has high rates and is 1 of 10 developed countries with the highest number of preterm births [10]. Preterm birth can further be subdivided on the basis of gestational age: extremely preterm (<28 weeks), very preterm (28–32 weeks), and moderate or late preterm [32–37] completed weeks of gestation. Since decreasing gestational age is associated with increasing mortality, disability, and cost due to intensity of neonatal care, these subdivisions are important [7]. As stated before, the risk of adverse consequences declines with increasing gestational age [9]. There are a variety of causes of preterm birth which can be broadly classified into (1) provider initiated preterm birth (induction of labor or elective cesarean section) before 37 weeks of gestation for maternal or fetal indications, (2) spontaneous preterm labor with intact membranes, and (3) preterm rupture of the membranes (PPROM), irrespective of whether delivery is vaginal or by cesarean section [9]. Births that follow spontaneous labor and PPROM are together referred to as spontaneous preterm births. As indicated in most studies, approximately 25% of all preterm births occur for maternal or fetal indications [5]. The contributions of the causes of preterm birth to all preterm births differ by ethnic groups. PPROM most commonly is the cause of preterm birth in black women, but spontaneous preterm birth is most commonly caused by preterm labor in white women [11]. In most studies, about 50% of all preterm births follow spontaneous preterm labor, and approximately 30% of preterm births result from premature rupture of the membranes. Obstetric intervention or iatrogenic preterm birth explains much of the increase seen in preterm births [12, 13]. Also, prior spontaneous preterm delivery is strongly associated with recurrence in the current pregnancy. An early prior spontaneous preterm delivery is a better predictor of recurrence and is most strongly associated with subsequent early spontaneous preterm delivery [14].

Ananth et al. tried to explain the reasons for the increase in preterm births over the last two decades by using large United States vital statistics data and concluded that a large part of increase in preterm births is explained by indicated preterm births [15]. Also a considerable increase is associated with multiple births that occur due to the use of various assisted reproductive techniques. Demographic and socioeconomic factors associated with increased risk of preterm birth include ethnicity, the presence of indicators of low socioeconomic status, and extreme maternal age among other factors [9]. A country-based study conducted in Italy showed an association between preterm birth and certain maternal outcomes as BMI, employment, previous abortions, previous preterm delivery, and previous cesarean section [16]. Some researchers believe preterm labor to be a syndrome initiated by multiple mechanisms, including infection or inflammation, utero-placental ischemia or hemorrhage, stress, and other immunologically mediated processes [11, 17]. A more concise mechanism is difficult to establish in most cases; therefore factors linked with preterm birth have been analyzed to explain preterm labor. Since many of the risk factors result in systemic inflammation, increasing infection or inflammation pathway might explain some of the variance in increase in preterm births associated with multiple risk factors [18]. Maternal BMI is an important risk factor for preterm birth and is of public health importance independently. Some researchers have shown an increase in preterm birth with low BMI or BMI <18.5 kg/m^2 [19–21]. Others support an increase in provider initiated preterm birth with increasing BMI [22, 23]. Cole-Lewis et al. suggest that there is evidence that pregnancy-specific stress is associated with preterm birth. They examined this relationship by measuring pregnancy-specific stress measured in the second and third trimesters in 920 black and/or Latina young women. Their findings emphasize the importance of measuring pregnancy-specific stress across the pregnancy. The longitudinal change from the second to third trimesters was significantly associated with the length of gestation measured both as a dichotomous variable (preterm birth) and a continuous variable. The results of the Cole-Lewis et al. study indicate that change in pregnancy-specific stress between the second and third trimesters was significantly associated with increased risk of preterm delivery and shortened gestational age, even after adjusting for important biological, behavioral, psychological, and sociocultural risk factors [24]. **Figure 1** depicts the sequelae of preterm birth.

3. Race and ethnicity and low birth weight

There is a strong association between both growth restriction and prematurity in newborns in women who belong to various ethnic and racial groups. Reasons for this association are not clear. In the United States, the rate of preterm birth in black women is about twice that of women from most other racial or ethnic groups. Similarly, black women are three to four times more likely to give birth to a very early preterm infant as compared to other racial groups [5, 25]. Women from South Asia and especially the Indian subcontinent have very high rates of growth restriction and low birth weight. In the United States, among all the groups, in black women the relationship between gestational age at birth of an infant and a particular pregnancy outcome, that is, low birth weight due to preterm, is very high, and to date this very high-preterm birth rate in black women is mostly unexplained.

4. Low birth weight and gestational age at birth

Infants born weighing <2500 g who are either born too early, that is, preterm birth, or too small, that is, fetal growth restriction, are referred to as low birth weight (LBW). LBW is an established factor associated with increased risk of infant mortality and morbidity, also a recognized proxy for maternal health [26, 27]. Garcia et al. have shown that after controlling for maternal age, parity, smoking, and maternal BMI, a significant difference was noted in infant mean birth weights and gestational age and hence rate of preterm birth between British and Indian, Pakistani, and Bangladeshi infants. This study confirms the evidence that South Asian women typically give birth to infants of lower birth weight than white British women, and a large variance in birth weight can be explained by a shorter gestational age in Indian mothers as compared to white British mothers [28]. One of the success stories in the United States and other developed countries is the improved survival in very LBW infants over the last three and a half decades. The survival for infants weighing between 500 and 1000 g in 1975 was approximately 15%. At present, survival for the same group of infants is 80%. Improvement in survival for infants born weighing between 1000 and 2500 g is also impressive. Approximately 60% of neonatal mortality is seen in newborns weighing <1000 g when the distribution of neonatal mortality by birth weight group is looked at [5].

The distribution of newborn the decreased rate of LBW in the United States is not seen across all 50 states. Some places like Washington DC and other mostly relatively poor southern states currently have a much higher rate of LBW rate than that of the United States (7.1%). The latest 2017 Alabama Kids Count Data Book, noted mixed results Statewide for children from 2005 to 2015 [29]. In Tuscaloosa County, Alabama, though the number of LBW babies has decreased from 12.6% during the last 10 years, the percentage is still higher than the state average of 10%. Unfortunately, the improvement in infants weighing between 1000 and 2500 g is not due to improvement in factors related to increased gestational age or reduction in rate of preterm birth. Highly sophisticated instruments and techniques are responsible for survival of these low and very low birth weights, without improving the factors associated with low birth weight, for example, increased length of gestation.

There are several long-term outcomes associated with low birth weight. The most common among them are neurological outcomes such as blindness, cerebral palsy, deafness, and hydrocephaly and several severe respiratory difficulties because of the poor lung development due to a short gestation. As indicated before, the earlier the gestational age and lower birth weight, the greater the risk for all complications and especially cerebral palsy [5, 7].

5. Stillbirth and gestational age at birth

The relationship between stillbirth and LBW and hence gestational age at birth of the infant is not studied frequently [30]. In the United States, approximately half of all still births occur at <28 weeks of gestational age. The other one-third occurs between 28 and 36 weeks of gestation [31]. Therefore, somewhere between two-thirds and three-quarters of all still births are mostly LBW and preterm. Thus both fetal growth restriction and preterm birth are significant risk factors for still birth. The risk of stillbirth after 32 weeks of gestation increases with gestational age, and half of these late fetal deaths occur at term [32]. Rosenstein et al. [33] and other researchers have reported that the risk of stillbirth at term increases with gestational age from 2.1/10,000 ongoing pregnancies at 37 weeks of gestation up to 10.8/10,000 ongoing pregnancies at 42 weeks of gestation. Also, at each gestational age beyond 38 weeks of gestation, the mortality risk of expectant management is higher than the risk of delivery, thus 39 weeks of gestation, 12.9 compared to 8.8/10,000; 40 weeks of gestation, 14.9 compared with 9.5/10,000; and 41 weeks, 17.6 compared with 10.8/10,000.

6. Fetal growth restriction and gestational age at birth

One of the major purposes of antenatal care is assessment of fetal growth. Caregivers need to distinguish between fetuses which are smaller than expected growth in utero; while some fetuses are constitutionally small, others have failed to meet their growth potential, that is, they are growth restricted (small for gestational age). While in the United States and other affluent countries, severe growth restriction is not common, the consequence of it not being recognized may include severe morbidity and in some cases even perinatal death [34]. According to the

Child Health Epidemiology Reference Group (CHERG) dataset which uses INTERGROWTH-21st standard, in 2012, an estimated 23.3 million or 19.3% infants were born small for gestational age in low- and middle-income countries [35]. Among these, 11.2 million were term and not LBW, 10.7 million were term and LBW, and 1.5 million were preterm. Also, in these low- or middle-income countries, an estimated 606,500 neonatal deaths were attributed to infants born too small for gestational age, 21.9% of all neonatal deaths. The prevalence in South Asia was highest. About 34% and approximately 26 of neonatal deaths were due to infants born too small for gestational age or growth restricted. Thus, in low- and middle-income countries, about one in five infants is born small for gestational age (as compared to 16% among blacks and 9% SGA in 200 in the United States), and one in four deaths is among such infants [36]. Growth restriction in infants can be due to many factors including poor maternal nutrition, maternal infections, congenital defects, smoking, and placental conditions [36]. SGA can also arise from genetic predisposition to small size. The genetic and constitutional contributions to SGA are generally small relative to the other factors mentioned above, particularly in low- and middle-income contexts. Infant survival strategies should direct resources toward leading causes of infant and child mortality, with attention focusing on infectious and neonatal causes. More rapid decrease from 2010 to 2015 will require accelerated reduction for most common causes of death, particularly, preterm and growth-restriction complications. Last but not least, gathering of high-quality data and enhanced estimation methods will be very useful for future estimates [37].

7. Chronic diseases and low birth weight and gestational age

Recently there have been many studies on the relation of LBW and gestational age at birth to the development of long-term chronic conditions, such as hypertension, diabetes, and heart disease. Termed as the Barker hypothesis, proposed in 1990 by the British epidemiologist David Barker that intrauterine growth retardation, low birth weight, and premature birth have a causal relationship to the origins of hypertension, coronary heart disease, and noninsulin-dependent diabetes [38]. Although its existence is controversial, it is supported by several epidemiological studies [39, 40].

8. Summary

The important pregnancy outcomes associated with gestational age at birth include both fetal and neonatal deaths, postnatal death, and short-term morbidities such as the respiratory distress syndrome and necrotizing enterocolitis. The long-term morbidities such as deafness, blindness, hydrocephaly, mental retardation, and cerebral palsy are among other chronic diseases discussed before. Many investigators use preterm birth (associated with gestational age) and growth restriction as an intermediate outcome measure for serious morbidity or mortality, that is, the goals of reducing growth retardation, preterm delivery, or length of gestational age are worthwhile only if they reflect reduction in morbidity and mortality. Thus, in some circumstances, if handicap or death is avoided, delivering an infant early is not the worst of all possible outcomes.

Author details

Yasmin H. Neggers

Address all correspondence to: yneggers@ches.ua.edu

Department of Human Nutrition, The University of Alabama, Tuscaloosa, AL, USA

References

[1] MedlinePlus. The National Institutes of health/ U.S. Library of Medicine. Available from: http://Medlineplus.gov/ency/article/002367.htm

[2] Carlos WA. The newborn infant. In: Kliegman RM, Staton BF, Geme JW, Schor NF editors. Nelson Textbook of Pediatrics. 20th ed. Philadelphia, PA: Elsevier; 2016. (Chapter 94)

[3] Goldenberg RL. Factors influencing perinatal outcomes. Annals of the New York Academy of Sciences. 2004;**1038**:227-234

[4] Hack M, Fanaroff AA. Outcomes of children of extremely low birth weight and gestational age in the 1990's. Early Human Development. 1999;**53**:193-218

[5] Goldenberg RL, Culhane JF. Low birthweight in the United States. American Journal of Clinical Nutrition. 2007;**85**(Suppl):584s-590s

[6] Neggers YH. The relationship between preterm birth and underweight in Asian women. Reproductive Toxicology. 2015;**56**:170-174

[7] Mathew TJ, Driscoll AK. Trends in infant mortality in the United States, 2005-2014. Available from: http://www.cdc.gov/nchs/products/databriefs/db279.htm [Accessed September 21, 2017]

[8] Riddle CA, Harper S, Kaufman JS. JAMA Pediatrics. Trends in differences in US mortality rates between black and white infants. 2017;**171**(9):911-912

[9] Platt MJ. Outcomes in preterm infants. PubMed Health. 2014;**128**:399-403

[10] Blencowe H, Cousens S, Chou D, Moller AB, Narwal R, Alder A, et al. National, regional, and worldwide estimates of preterm birth rates in the year 2010 with time trends since 1990 for selected countries: a systematic analysis and implications. Lancet. 2012;**379**:2162-2172

[11] Goldenberg RL, Culhane JF, Iams JD, Romero R. Epidemiology and causes of preterm birth. Lancet. 2008;**371**:75-84

[12] Raisanen S, Gissler M, Kramer M, Heinonen S. Contribution of risk factors to extremely, very and moderately preterm births-register-based analysis of 1,390,742 singleton births. PLoS One. 2013;**894**:e60660

[13] Lisnokova S, Hutcheon JA, Joseph KS. Temporal trends in neonatal outcome following iatrogenic preterm delivery. BMC Pregnancy &Childbirth. 2011;**11**:39. DOI: 10.1186/1471-2393-11-39

[14] Mercer BM, Goldenberg RL, Moawad AH, Meis PJ, Iams JD, Das AF, et al. The preterm prediction study: Effect of gestational age and cause of preterm birth on subsequent obstetrics outcome. American Journal of Obstetrics and Gynecology. 1999;**181**(5 Pt 1):1216-1221

[15] Ananth CV, Joseph KS, Oyelese Y, Demisse K, Vintzileos AM. Trends in preterm birth and perinatal mortality amng singletons: United States, 1989 through 2000. Obstetrics & Gynecology. 2005;**105**:1084-1091

[16] Di Renzo GC, Giardina I, Rosati A, Graziano C, Torricelli M, Petraglia F. Maternal risk factors for preterm birth: a country-based population analysis. European Journal of Obstetrics & Gynecology and Reproductive Biology 2011;**159**:342-346

[17] Romero R, Espinoza J, Kusanovic JP, et al. The preterm parturition syndrome. British Journal of Obstetrics and Gynaecology. 2006;**113**:17-42

[18] Goldenberg RL, Culhane JF. Preprenancy health status and risk of preterm delivery. Archives of Pediatrics & Adolescent Medicine. 2005;**159**:89-90

[19] Neggers YH, Goldenberg RL, Cliver SP, Hauth J. The relationship between psychosocial profile, health practices and pregnancy outcomes. Acta Obstetricia et Gynecologica Scandinavica. 2006;**85**:277-285

[20] Hendler I, Goldenberg RL, Mercer BM. The preterm prediction study: Association between maternal body mass index and spontaneous and indicated preterm birth. American Journal of Obstetrics and Gynecology. 2005;**192**:882-886

[21] Smith GC, Shah I, Pell JP, Crossley JA, Dobbie R. Maternal obesity in early pregnancy and risk of spontaneous and elective preterm deliveries: A trospective cohort study. American Journal of Public Health. 2007;**97**:157-162

[22] Torolini MR, Betran AP, Daher S. Maternal BMI and preterm birth: A systematic review of the literature with meta-analysis. Fetal & Neonatal Medicine. 2009;**22**:957-970

[23] McDonald SD, Han Z, Mulla S, Beyene J. Overweight and obesity in mother and risk of preterm birth and low birth weight infants: Systematic review. British Medical Journal. 2010;**341**:c428

[24] Cole-Lewis H, Kershaw TS, Earnshaw VA, Yonkers KA, Haiqun LA, Ickovics JR. Pregnancy-specific stress, preterm birth, and gestational age among high-risk women. Health Psychology. 2014;**33**(9):1033-1045

[25] Schieve LA, Handler A. Preterm delivery and perinatal death among Black and White infants in Chicago-area perinatal registry. Obstetrics & Gynecology. 1996;**88**:356-363

[26] Institute of Health Economics. Determinants and Prevention of Low Birth Weight: A Synopsis of the Evidence. Alberta, Canada: Institute of Health Economics; 2008

[27] Joshi KJ, Sochaliya KM, Shrivastav AV. A hospital based study on the prevalence of low birth weight in new born babies and its relation to maternal health factors. International Journal of Research in Medical Sciences. 2014;**3**:4-8

[28] Garcia R, Ali N, Guppy A, Griffith M Randhawa G. Differences in pregnancy gestation period and mean birthweight in infants born to Indian, Pakistani, Bangladeshi and white British mother in Luton, UK. BMJ Open. 2017;**7**:e017139. DOI: 1136/bmjopen-2017-017139

[29] Mann R. Kids Count Data Center. Voices for Alabama's Children. The Annie Casey Foundation. 2017. Available from: http://www.alavoices.org

[30] Goldenberg RL, Kirby R, Culhane JF. Stillbirth: A review. Journal of Maternal-Fetal & Neonatal Medicine. 2004;**16**:79-94

[31] Goldenberg RL, Koski JF, Boyd BW, Cutter GR, Nelson KG. Fetal deaths in Alabama 1974-1983: A birth weight specific analysis. Obstetrics & Gynecology. 1987;**70**:831-835

[32] Reddy UM, Ko CW, Willinger M. maternal age and risk of stillbirth throughout pregnancy in the United States. American Journal of Obstetrics & Gynecology. 2006;**195**:764-770

[33] Rosenstein MG, Cheng YW, Snowden JM, Nicholson JM, Caughey AB. Risk of stillbirth and infant death stratified by gestational age. Obstetrics & Gynecology. 2012;**120**(1):76-82

[34] Andrew CG, Breeze C, Lees C. Prediction and perinatal outcomes of fetal growth. Seminars in Fetal & Neonatal Medicine. 2007;**12**:383-397

[35] Lee A, Kozuki N, Cousens S, Stevens GA, Blencowe H, Silveira M, et al. Etimates of burden and consequences of infants born small for gestational age low and middle income countries with INTERGROWTH- 21 standard: Analysis of CHERG datasets. British Medical Journal. 2017;**358**:3677-3702

[36] Katz J, Wu LA, Mullany LC, Coles CL, Anne C, Kozuki N. Prevalence of small for gestational age and its mortality risk varies by choice of birth weight for gestation reference population. PLoS One. 2014;**9**(3):e92074

[37] Liu L, Cousens S, Perin J, Scott S, Lawn JE, Rudan I, et al. Global, regional, and national causes of child mortality: Van updated systematic analysis for 2010 with time trends since 2000. Lancet. 2012;**379**:2151-2161

[38] Barker DJ. Fetal origins of cardiovascular disease. Annals of Medicine. 1999;**31**(Suppl): S54-S58

[39] Calkins K, Devaskar SU. Fetal origins of adult disease. Current Problems in Pediatric and Adolescent Health Care. 2011;**41**(6):158-176

[40] Robison JS Moore VM, Owens JA Mcmillen IC. Origins of fetal growth restriction. Obstetrics & Gynecology. 2000;**92**:13-19

Chapter 3

Smoking: An Important Environmental Risk Factor in Pregnancy

Qing Xia, Jing Yang and Qiuqin Tang

Additional information is available at the end of the chapter

http://dx.doi.org/10.5772/intechopen.72209

Abstract

It is generally recognized that smoking has been one of the most public health disorders around the world. Nowadays, more and more studies have proved that smoking during pregnancy is responsible for both maternal and fetal health disorders along with several general health effects. It may lead to various kinds of pregnancy illness and cause risk to the fetus during perinatal stage. After birth, this behavior can also have harmful influences on neonates, and even on children. However, smoking during pregnancy has several adverse effects, the molecular mechanism of it remains unclear. Recently, some studies have proved that it is associated with aberrant epigenetic modifications. All of these remind us that more attention should be paid to maternal cigarette smoking, and more studies should be carried out to confirm the effects and investigate the molecular mechanisms. In this chapter, a brief review is given on the perinatal effects and long-term influences of maternal and passive smoking. We also briefly clarify the epigenetic mechanisms underlying the adverse effects of passive smoking during pregnancy.

Keywords: smoking, passive smoking, pregnancy, perinatal effects, effects on neonates

1. Introduction

It is generally recognized that smoking has been one of the most public health problems around the world because it is widespread and harmful. According to the statistics, there are over 1.2 billion smokers all over the world, and nearly 4.9 million people are dying from smoking [1].

As an invisible cause of death, smoking during pregnancy is responsible for both maternal and fetal health disorders including miscarriage and congenital abnormalities along with several general health effects (e.g., cardiovascular disease, respiratory disease, cancer) [2, 3].

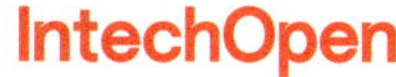

The substances contained in cigarettes may cause harm to the fetus. Among those substances, two compounds are especially harmful: nicotine and carbon monoxide. Nicotine is highly addicted. It is well studied that nicotine is a carcinogen and extremely toxic in tobacco leaves, which results in many responses such as increasing heart rate and blood pressure. Meanwhile, carbon monoxide can also lead to fetal hypoxia. Thus, the infant whose mother smokes has a higher perinatal morbidity and mortality. Also, there are many other harmful compounds such as arsenic, formaldehyde, lead, uranium, and ammonia.

This chapter introduces the great harm done to the developing fetus resulting from maternal smoking and passive smoking, which creates problems that will prevail not only during the pregnancy but also long after parturition.

2. Perinatal effects

2.1. Preterm birth

It has been a significant global problem with more than 10% of babies suffering from it. Preterm birth or other relevant disorders lead to death of a million children each year worldwide [4]. Several factors can lead to premature birth, for example, underlying infection or some anatomical considerations. Besides, smoking during pregnancy is also an important factor that may cause preterm birth. Since nicotine exposure leads to several complications of pregnancy and birth, the risk for preterm birth is higher among women who smoke during pregnancy. It is shown that the probability of preterm birth is over 1% higher for women who smoke during pregnancy than others [5]. There are several elements contributing to the alteration of steroid hormone production and changes of the responses to oxytocin such as hypoxia resulting from carbon monoxide and vasoconstriction resulting from nicotine [6].

Using Taiwan Birth Cohort to explore the effects of maternal smoking on birth outcomes, Ko et al. [7] found that maternal smoking is associated with preterm delivery. The incidences of preterm birth of mothers who smoked during the different pregnancy stages increased with the number of cigarettes smoked daily, which was especially significant among those who smoked more than 20 cigarettes/day.

Unlike other unavoidable factors for preterm birth, tobacco smoking is an environmental exposure which can be easily eliminated, and even short behavioral interventions can be effective.

2.2. Ectopic pregnancy

Transport of the fertilized egg through the fallopian tube is controlled by ciliary beating and smooth muscle contractility [8]. Ectopic pregnancy (tubal pregnancy), or eccyesis, is a complication of pregnancy in which the embryo attached outside the uterus [9]. Ectopic pregnancy in the fallopian tubes are more common among smoking women as nicotine or other substances of cigarettes may lead to the turnover of altered epithelial cell in the fallopian tube and result in the dysfunction of fallopian tube. Several risk factors of damaging or killing cilia can result from smoking, thus increasing the time for the embryo to reach the uterus. The embryo, which cannot reach the uterus in time, will implant itself inside the fallopian tube, causing the ectopic pregnancy [10]. Besides ectopic pregnancy, cigarette smoking during pregnancy also leads to other human reproduction disorders such as spontaneous abortion and infertility [11].

2.3. Premature rupture of membranes (PROM)

PROM, also known as rupture of membranes occurring in pregnancy, refers to breakage of the amniotic sac. Commonly, it is called breaking of the mother's water [12]. There is amniotic fluid surrounding and protecting the fetus in the uterus contained in the sac (including two membranes, the chorion and the amnion). When rupture occurs, the fluid leaks out of the uterus through the vagina. Fetal membranes will be likely to be broken because they become weak and fragile. This change is usually a normal process that happens along with the body preparing for labor or delivery. However, this will become a problem when premature birth occurs. Cigarette smoking during pregnancy leads to the abnormal weakness of fetal membranes by the factors of cell death and poor assembly of collagen, and even breakdown of collagen [13].

2.4. Pregnancy-induced hypertension and preeclampsia

Similar with overweight, smoking during pregnancy is shown as an inverse risk factor for hypertensive disorders of pregnancy such as pregnancy-induced hypertension and preeclampsia. Studies demonstrate that, compared with women of normal weight, pregnancy-induced hypertension and gestational hypertension are more common among overweight women, especially in overweight women who smoke. The risk for hypertensive disorders increases 2–3 times among overweight and obese women [14, 15], which reflects an independent effects of obesity or smoking habits on the hypertensive disorders.

On the contrary, there is an inverse association that smoking in women of normal weight has potential effect of decreasing the risk of pregnancy-induced hypertensive disorders. Barquiel et al. [16] found that prepregnancy overweight or obesity and excess gestational weight gain are all associated with pregnancy-induced hypertensive disorders. However, there is no clinical proof of the potentially positive effect of nicotine exposure on hypertensive disorders. It is hypothesized that the combustion of tobacco products circulating angiogenic proteins, which could be released through carbon monoxide [6, 17].

2.5. Fetal growth restriction

Several studies have demonstrated that fetuses with prenatal nicotine exposure have lower birth weight than their peers [18, 19], and the findings are consistent with intrauterine growth restriction [20, 21]. Imaging examination shows that this growth restriction affects brain, kidney, lung, and other lean and fatty tissues. Overall fetal volume and placental volume are also decreased, which may result in embryo damage and miscarriages, thus increasing the infant mortality [22, 23]. This effect is found to be dose-dependent. There is a decreased birth weight by an average of 2.8 g for each additional pack of cigarette smoked during pregnancy [23].

According to a large nationwide birth cohort study in Japan, Suzuki et al. [24] found that maternal smoking during pregnancy can lead to lower birth weight by 125–136 g.

The mechanism of fetal growth restriction is under debate. Several initial studies demonstrated that fetal hypoxia is induced by the carbon monoxide or other combustion products [6, 25]. However, it is observed that using electronic cigarettes also results in fetal growth restriction, making this view seems less likely [22]. Numerous researchers agree that smoking during pregnancy significantly increases the resistance of placental blood flow, which is associated with fetal growth restriction [26, 27]. It may be seen that fetal growth restriction results from nicotine, which leads to the vasoconstriction. While there is another theory proposing that decreased supply of amino acids contributes to fetal growth restriction. Nicotine exposure blocks the cholinergic receptor and impairs amino acid transport [28], while the hypoxia resulting from carbon monoxide also limits the transport of amino acids.

3. Effects on neonates

3.1. Sudden infant death syndrome (SIDS)

SIDS is one of the main reasons for death among healthy infants [29]. It is defined as the sudden death of 1-year-old neonates. SIDS usually occurs with no struggle, no noise produced, and always happens between 00:00 and 09:00 during children's sleep [30]. SIDS seems to occur when a neonate has an underlying biological vulnerability, such as premature infants or low-birth-weight infants, or has problems in the part of the brain [31]. Studies show that SIDS rates are higher in infants with fetal growth restriction resulting from prenatal nicotine exposure [32]. The study of Zhang and Wang [33] also suggested that maternal smoking could increase the risk of SIDS, and it was dose-dependent. Mitchell and Milerad [34] discovered that the exposure of the fetus to tobacco is associated with SIDS. They also suggested that if maternal smoking is avoided, about one-third of SIDS deaths might have been hold back. However, until now, no one knows the exact cause of SIDS, and the mechanism that how prenatal nicotine exposure leads to SIDS remains unclear.

3.2. Future obesity and endocrine imbalance

Similar to fetal restriction, studies proved that prenatal smoking could affect growth patterns over the long term, with height deficits documented in childhood through to adulthood [35]. Disproportionate weight gain opposite to fetal growth restriction is considered to be associated with the infant's self-regulation of food intake after birth, as small-for-date babies take more milk than large-for-date babies, suggested by Ounsted's study [36]. A recent study has proposed that despite birthing with lower weights, children of mothers who smoke during pregnancy tend to be overweight [37, 38], and such an effect will last for a lifetime [39, 40]. It is noted that alterations in ghrelin concentrations are likely to be involved [41]. Thus, the offspring of smoking mothers takes more risk of suffering from type 2 diabetes [42, 43].

Alternatively, endocrine imbalances could occur at critical developmental periods. Studies point out negative effects of prenatal smoking on reproductive system. The menarche may be earlier in females exposed to nicotine prenatally [25]. In males, analysis of semen samples points out that prenatal nicotine exposure results in poor semen quality and decreased sperm count [44, 45]. This indicates that such long-term health consequences are not confined to one generation, but also continued to impair the health of a future generation.

3.3. Respiratory tract infections and compromised lung function

Maternal smoking can also influence fetal lung development and lung function. The embryonic immune function will have over reaction to certain substances, thus producing antibodies, which are easy to cause allergic diseases after the baby was born. Pulmonary function testing demonstrates that the impaired lung function of children is associated with the exposure to nicotine prenatally [46, 47]. Compared with their peers, the incidents of respiratory tract infections and compromised lung function (e.g., asthma or wheezing) increased [48, 49], as a result of developmental anomalies in the lung caused by nicotine. These changes will impair the gas-exchange ability of the pulmonary parenchyma, leading to a directly increased amount of work for respiration [50]. In addition, Hayatbakhsh et al. [51] proved that the bad effects on the growth and development of the respiratory tract may continue into adulthood.

3.4. Congenital heart defects and hypertension

As is shown that nicotine increases placental vascular resistance [52, 53], children with maternal nicotine exposures tend to have a greater risk of hypertension throughout the whole life [54, 55]. Further studies show that women who smoke during pregnancy put their fetus at a higher risk of birth defects, especially congenital heart defects than their peers [56, 57]. Using an epidemiological case-control study, Kuciene and Dulskiene [58] collected the information on potential risk factors of newborns' health. They chose 261 newborns with congenital heart septal defects and 1122 randomly selected newborns without any defects. They found that smoking during pregnancy can increase the risk of congenital heart septal defects in infants.

However, the effect of smoking during pregnancy on the progeny of hypertension is not clear. De Jonge et al. [59] found that the association between smoking during pregnancy and the risk of hypertension in the offspring are largely determined by weight, and the mechanisms in utero remain unknown.

3.5. Brain function

Since there are many toxic chemicals in tobacco, smoking during pregnancy can restrict the head growth, change the structure and function of the brain, and have lifelong bad effects on the fetal brains. In addition to the direct impact of the chemical composition, evidence suggests that smokers are more susceptible to depression and refuse to take health promoting actions. To be specific, smokers will not receive prenatal care timely and recognize their pregnancies later [60]. Along with the adverse effects of nicotine on the fetal brain, children of smokers are more likely to have learning disorders or behavioral problems. El Marroun et al. [60] proved that smoking during pregnancy is associated with brain dysfunction of children. They found that maternal cigarette smoking can lead to smaller brain volumes, smaller cortical gray and white matter volumes of children, and these children will also have thinner superior frontal, superior parietal, lateral occipital, and precentral cortices, and show more behavioral and emotional problems.

In conclusion, smoking during pregnancy can cause bad effects on the growth of the fetal head and influence the normal brain function [61]. However, the mechanisms of how these bad effects happen on the fetus need more research.

4. Effects of passive smoking

We all know that maternal active smoking is harmful to pregnant women and the fetus; however, more and more studies have showed that passive smoking is also a hidden threat [62]. Ohida et al. [63] demonstrated that passive smoking could make pregnant women suffer from sleep disturbance, because nicotine affected the central nervous system, kept people awake, and increased the sleep latency, reduced both total sleep time and REM sleep. Qiu et al. [64] have found that passive smoking can lead to preterm birth. However, when they stratified the data by gestational age, they also found that passive smoking was strongly associated with very preterm birth (<32 weeks of gestation) but not with moderate preterm birth (32–36 weeks of gestation), and the risk of very preterm birth is increased when the time of the exposure to tobacco is increased.

In recent years, many anti-smoking activities have been carried out in public places to prevent nonsmoking women and children who suffer from passive smoking. However, bad effects of passive smoking on pregnant women have not been widely publicized because they are less clear, and many people are still not aware of them. So more studies should be carried out to ensure bad outcomes of pregnant women associated with passive smoking.

5. The epigenetic mechanism of adverse effect of smoking during pregnancy

Several studies have demonstrated that smoking during pregnancy takes effects through epigenetic mechanisms, just like other environmental factors. Knopik et al. [65] proved that smoking during pregnancy can change the process of DNA methylation and disrupt miRNA expression. They deemed that maternal cigarette smoking was associated with incorrect DNA methylation patterns, which were important for the health of the embryo, and it could also lead to the aberrant expression of miRNA. Therefore, many biological processes would be disturbed. Suter et al. found that smoking during pregnancy is associated with aberrant placental epigenome-wide DNA methylation and gene expression, including changes in promoter methylation of placental *CYP1A1*, which are related to *CYP1A1* gene expression and fetal growth restriction. They also suggested that smoking during pregnancy is concerned with altered site-specific CpG methylation which is necessary for important changes in gene expression, which ensure proper growth and development [66]. Lee et al. [67] demonstrated that smoking during pregnancy may change the DNA methylation of the offspring reproducibly, which may last for many years, even into adolescence.

Although many facts show that smoking during pregnancy has many bad effects in terms of epigenetics, we still cannot figure out the specific process of it. Therefore, more studies should be done to increase the understanding of mechanisms involved.

6. Anti-smoking measures

Since smoking during pregnancy can lead to many bad effects on pregnant women, the fetus, and newborns, increasing awareness of the consequences of smoking during pregnancy among women is obviously very important. However, participants were not fully aware of the bad outcomes of smoking during pregnancy [68]. Koren [69] showed that about 25–30% of women smoke at the beginning of the pregnancy. Many pregnant women had given up smoking for the health of the fetus; however, some of them remained smoking during pregnancy. The study indicated that except those psychosocial factors, nicotine addiction is widely acknowledged as the main reason of smoking cessation failures. So, they put forward a smoking cessation therapy called nicotine replacement therapy. It used nicotine patches, gum, or intranasal preparations to help people quit smoking, and was superior to placebo.

For pregnant women who are already smoking, smoking cessation is necessary because smoking during pregnancy can damage the health of the fetus. The adverse effects of smoking may be attenuated if mothers quit or reduce the cigarette consumption during pregnancy, because cigarette quitting can increase the use of multivitamin and decrease the consumption of caffeine. However, smoking cessation in early pregnancy may have negative impacts, because it can increase high caloric intake, and high caloric intake in the first trimester may have bad effects on maternal and child health [70]. In general, behavioral therapies and patient education should be recommended as first-line therapy for smoking cessation. However, if someone fails to quit smoking, nicotine replacement therapy can be attempted as an adjuvant treatment [71].

7. Conclusion

As one of the most important environmental factors that influence the health of human, smoking can lead to a series of health problems, and smoking during pregnancy will have a great impact on the fetus (**Figure 1**). Prenatal nicotine exposure affects the mother and fetus in many ways, such as respiratory tract, lung, cardiovascular, brain, and leads to many chronic

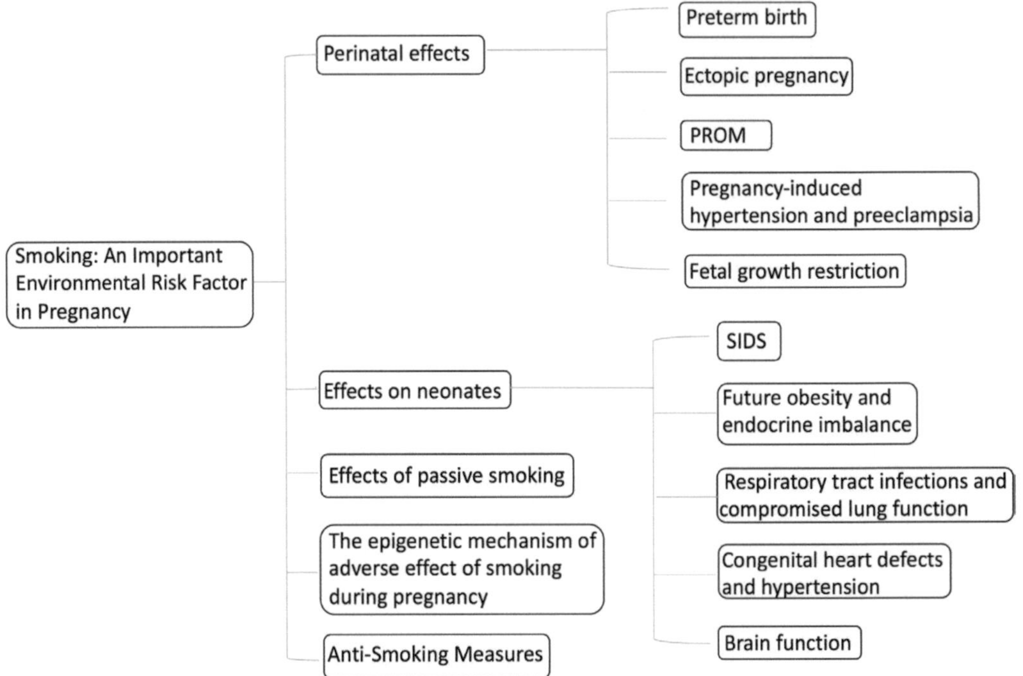

Figure 1. Schematic representation of smoking as an important environmental risk factor in pregnancy.

diseases. Longitudinal studies have shown that the vast majority of these effects (e.g., health effects, learning disorders, or behavioral problems) will last for the whole life, and have profound influences on the growth of children. Moreover, not only the active smoking but also the passive smoking can affect the health of the fetus greatly (**Figure 1**).

Studies have pointed out that nicotine exposure has the most harmful effects during the third trimester. This provides a remedial opportunity for these smoking mothers to improve the status of the pregnancy and their children's health for life. In view of the widespread use of tobacco and the harmful effects of nicotine, more anti-measures should be carried out to create a smoke-free environment for pregnant women, and the education related to the harmful effects of cigarette smoking during pregnancy should be carried on and the expectant mothers should be advised to quit smoking at least during their pregnancy. Also, more effective therapies should be explored to help pregnant women quit smoking. Nowadays, more and more people pay attention to the environmental factors that can affect the health of pregnant women and the fetus. We believe further studies will provide more details of the effects of nicotine, carbon monoxide, and other substances of the cigarette, which may contribute to creating a greater sense of urgency about smoking cessation in patients. Also, we should explore more accurate epigenetic mechanisms to help us better understand how those chemicals affect offspring, so that we can find better treatments for the affected children.

Author details

Qing Xia[1,2], Jing Yang[1,2] and Qiuqin Tang[3*]

*Address all correspondence to: t19871004@sina.com

1 State Key Laboratory of Reproductive Medicine, Institute of Toxicology, Nanjing Medical University, Nanjing, China

2 Key Laboratory of Modern Toxicology of Ministry of Education, School of Public Health, Nanjing Medical University, Nanjing, China

3 Department of Obstetrics, Obstetrics and Gynecology Hospital Affiliated to Nanjing Medical University, Nanjing Maternity and Child Health Hospital, Nanjing, China

References

[1] Chronic Periodontitis—Prevention, Diagnosis and Treatment: A Systematic Review. SBU Systematic Review Summaries. Stockholm; 2004

[2] Price JF, Mowbray PI, Lee AJ, Rumley A, Lowe GD, Fowkes FG. Relationship between smoking and cardiovascular risk factors in the development of peripheral arterial disease and coronary artery disease: Edinburgh Artery Study. European Heart Journal. 1999;**20**(5):344-353

[3] Armani C, Landini jr L, Leone A. Molecular and biochemical changes of the cardiovascular system due to smoking exposure. Current Pharmaceutical Design. 2009;**15**(10):1038-1053

[4] Blencowe H, Cousens S, Oestergaard MZ, Chou D, Moller AB, Narwal R, et al. National, regional, and worldwide estimates of preterm birth rates in the year 2010 with time trends since 1990 for selected countries: A systematic analysis and implications. Lancet. 2012;**379**(9832):2162-2172

[5] Anderka M, Romitti PA, Sun L, Druschel C, Carmichael S, Shaw G, et al. Patterns of tobacco exposure before and during pregnancy. Acta Obstetricia et Gynecologica Scandinavica. 2010;**89**(4):505-514

[6] Wikstrom AK, Stephansson O, Cnattingius S. Tobacco use during pregnancy and preeclampsia risk: Effects of cigarette smoking and snuff. Hypertension. 2010;**55**(5):1254-1259

[7] Ko TJ, Tsai LY, Chu LC, Yeh SJ, Leung C, Chen CY, et al. Parental smoking during pregnancy and its association with low birth weight, small for gestational age, and preterm birth offspring: A birth cohort study. Pediatrics and Neonatology. 2014;**55**(1):20-27

[8] Lindblom B, Hamberger L, Ljung B. Contractile patterns of isolated oviductal smooth muscle under different hormonal conditions. Fertility and sterility. 1980;**33**(3):283-287

[9] Kirk E, Bottomley C, Bourne T. Diagnosing ectopic pregnancy and current concepts in the management of pregnancy of unknown location. Human Reproduction Update. 2014; **20**(2):250-261

[10] Lyons RA, Saridogan E, Djahanbakhch O. The reproductive significance of human fallopian tube cilia. Human Reproduction Update. 2006;**12**(4):363-372

[11] Stillman RJ, Rosenberg MJ, Sachs BP. Smoking and reproduction. Fertility and Sterility. 1986;**46**(4):545-566

[12] Practice bulletins No. 139: Premature rupture of membranes. Obstetrics and Gynecology. 2013;**122**(4):918-930

[13] Okunade KS, Oluwole AA, Adegbesan-Omilabu MA. A study on the association between low maternal serum magnesium level and preterm labour. Advances in Medicine. 2014;**2014**:704875

[14] Bodnar LM, Ness RB, Markovic N, Roberts JM. The risk of preeclampsia rises with increasing prepregnancy body mass index. Annals of Epidemiology. 2005;**15**(7):475-482

[15] Catov JM, Ness RB, Kip KE, Olsen J. Risk of early or severe pre-eclampsia related to pre-existing conditions. International Journal of Epidemiology. 2007;**36**(2):412-419

[16] Barquiel B, Herranz L, Grande C, Castro-Dufourny I, Llaro M, Parra P, et al. Body weight, weight gain and hyperglycaemia are associated with hypertensive disorders of pregnancy in women with gestational diabetes. Diabetes & Metabolism. 2014;**40**(3):204-210

[17] Levine RJ, Maynard SE, Qian C, Lim KH, England LJ, KF Y, et al. Circulating angiogenic factors and the risk of preeclampsia. The New England Journal of Medicine. 2004;**350**(7):672-683

[18] Fried PA, O'Connell CM. A comparison of the effects of prenatal exposure to tobacco, alcohol, cannabis and caffeine on birth size and subsequent growth. Neurotoxicology and Teratology. 1987;**9**(2):79-85

[19] Slotkin TA. Fetal nicotine or cocaine exposure: Which one is worse? The Journal of Pharmacology and Experimental Therapeutics. 1998;**285**(3):931-945

[20] Mitchell EA, Thompson JM, Robinson E, Wild CJ, Becroft DM, Clark PM, et al. Smoking, nicotine and tar and risk of small for gestational age babies. Acta Paediatrica. 2002; **91**(3):323-328

[21] Jaddoe VW, Verburg BO, de Ridder MA, Hofman A, Mackenbach JP, Moll HA, et al. Maternal smoking and fetal growth characteristics in different periods of pregnancy: The generation R study. American Journal of Epidemiology. 2007;**165**(10):1207-1215

[22] Baba S, Wikstrom AK, Stephansson O, Cnattingius S. Changes in snuff and smoking habits in Swedish pregnant women and risk for small for gestational age births. BJOG: An International Journal of Obstetrics and Gynaecology. 2013;**120**(4):456-462

[23] Harrod CS, Reynolds RM, Chasan-Taber L, Fingerlin TE, Glueck DH, Brinton JT, et al. Quantity and timing of maternal prenatal smoking on neonatal body composition: The Healthy Start study. The Journal of Pediatrics. 2014;**165**(4):707-712

[24] Suzuki K, Shinohara R, Sato M, Otawa S, Yamagata Z. Association between maternal smoking during pregnancy and birth weight: An appropriately adjusted model from the Japan environment and Children's study. Journal of Epidemiology. 2016;**26**(7):371-377

[25] Ernst M, Moolchan ET, Robinson ML. Behavioral and neural consequences of prenatal exposure to nicotine. Journal of the American Academy of Child and Adolescent Psychiatry. 2001;**40**(6):630-641

[26] Kho EM, North RA, Chan E, Stone PR, Dekker GA, McCowan LM, et al. Changes in Doppler flow velocity waveforms and fetal size at 20 weeks gestation among cigarette smokers. BJOG: An International Journal of Obstetrics and Gynaecology. 2009;**116**(10):1300-1306

[27] Pringle PJ, Geary MP, Rodeck CH, Kingdom JC, Kayamba-Kay's S, Hindmarsh PC. The influence of cigarette smoking on antenatal growth, birth size, and the insulin-like growth factor axis. The Journal of Clinical Endocrinology and Metabolism. 2005;**90**(5): 2556-2562

[28] Sastry BV. Placental toxicology: Tobacco smoke, abused drugs, multiple chemical interactions, and placental function. Reproduction, Fertility, and Development. 1991; **3**(4):355-372

[29] Adams SM, Good MW, Defranco GM. Sudden infant death syndrome. American Family Physician. 2009;**79**(10):870-874

[30] Kinney HC, Thach BT. The sudden infant death syndrome. The New England Journal of Medicine. 2009;**361**(8):795-805

[31] Sudden Infant Death Syndrome (SIDS). American Family Physician. 2015;**91**(11):Online.

[32] Sullivan FM, Barlow SM. Review of risk factors for sudden infant death syndrome. Paediatric and Perinatal Epidemiology. 2001;**15**(2):144-200

[33] Zhang K, Wang X. Maternal smoking and increased risk of sudden infant death syndrome: A meta-analysis. Legal Medicine. 2013;**15**(3):115-121

[34] Mitchell EA, Milerad J. Smoking and the sudden infant death syndrome. Reviews on Environmental Health. 2006;**21**(2):81-103

[35] Butler NR, Goldstein H. Smoking in pregnancy and subsequent child development. British Medical Journal. 1973;**4**(5892):573-575

[36] Ounsted M, Sleigh G. The infant's self-regulation of food intake and weight gain. Difference in metabolic balance after growth constraint or acceleration in utero. Lancet. 1975;**1**(7922):1393-1397

[37] Toschke AM, Koletzko B, Slikker W Jr, Hermann M, von Kries R. Childhood obesity is associated with maternal smoking in pregnancy. European Journal of Pediatrics. 2002;**161**(8):445-448

[38] Bergmann KE, Bergmann RL, Von Kries R, Bohm O, Richter R, Dudenhausen JW, et al. Early determinants of childhood overweight and adiposity in a birth cohort study: Role of breast-feeding. International Journal of Obesity and Related Metabolic Disorders: Journal of the International Association for the Study of Obesity. 2003;**27**(2):162-172

[39] Oken E, Levitan EB, Gillman MW. Maternal smoking during pregnancy and child overweight: Systematic review and meta-analysis. International Journal of Obesity. 2008;**32**(2):201-210

[40] Haghighi A, Schwartz DH, Abrahamowicz M, Leonard GT, Perron M, Richer L, et al. Prenatal exposure to maternal cigarette smoking, amygdala volume, and fat intake in adolescence. JAMA Psychiatry. 2013;**70**(1):98-105

[41] Paslakis G, Buchmann AF, Westphal S, Banaschewski T, Hohm E, Zimmermann US, et al. Intrauterine exposure to cigarette smoke is associated with increased ghrelin concentrations in adulthood. Neuroendocrinology. 2014;**99**(2):123-129

[42] Syme C, Abrahamowicz M, Mahboubi A, Leonard GT, Perron M, Richer L, et al. Prenatal exposure to maternal cigarette smoking and accumulation of intra-abdominal fat during adolescence. Obesity. 2010;**18**(5):1021-1025

[43] Bruin JE, Gerstein HC, Holloway AC. Long-term consequences of fetal and neonatal nicotine exposure: A critical review. Toxicological Sciences: An Official Journal of the Society of Toxicology. 2010;**116**(2):364-374

[44] Storgaard L, Bonde JP, Ernst E, Spano M, Andersen CY, Frydenberg M, et al. Does smoking during pregnancy affect sons' sperm counts? Epidemiology. 2003;**14**(3):278-286

[45] Ravnborg TL, Jensen TK, Andersson AM, Toppari J, Skakkebaek NE, Jorgensen N. Prenatal and adult exposures to smoking are associated with adverse effects on reproductive hormones, semen quality, final height and body mass index. Human Reproduction. 2011;**26**(5):1000-1011

[46] Hollams EM, de Klerk NH, Holt PG, Sly PD. Persistent effects of maternal smoking during pregnancy on lung function and asthma in adolescents. American Journal of Respiratory and Critical Care Medicine. 2014;**189**(4):401-407

[47] Maritz GS, Harding R. Life-long programming implications of exposure to tobacco smoking and nicotine before and soon after birth: Evidence for altered lung development. International Journal of Environmental Research and Public Health. 2011;**8**(3):875-898

[48] Brown RW, Hanrahan JP, Castile RG, Tager IB. Effect of maternal smoking during pregnancy on passive respiratory mechanics in early infancy. Pediatric Pulmonology. 1995;**19**(1):23-28

[49] Sekhon HS, Keller JA, Benowitz NL, Spindel ER. Prenatal nicotine exposure alters pulmonary function in newborn rhesus monkeys. American Journal of Respiratory and Critical Care Medicine. 2001;**164**(6):989-994

[50] Klings ES, Safaya S, Adewoye AH, Odhiambo A, Frampton G, Lenburg M, et al. Differential gene expression in pulmonary artery endothelial cells exposed to sickle cell plasma. Physiological Genomics. 2005;**21**(3):293-298

[51] Hayatbakhsh MR, Sadasivam S, Mamun AA, Najman JM, Williams GM, O'Callaghan MJ. Maternal smoking during and after pregnancy and lung function in early adulthood: A prospective study. Thorax. 2009;**64**(9):810-814

[52] Machado Jde B, Plinio Filho VM, Petersen GO, Chatkin JM. Quantitative effects of tobacco smoking exposure on the maternal-fetal circulation. BMC Pregnancy and Childbirth. 2011;**11**:24

[53] Morrow RJ, Ritchie JW, Bull SB. Maternal cigarette smoking: The effects on umbilical and uterine blood flow velocity. American Journal of Obstetrics and Gynecology. 1988;**159**(5):1069-1071

[54] Oken E, Huh SY, Taveras EM, Rich-Edwards JW, Gillman MW. Associations of maternal prenatal smoking with child adiposity and blood pressure. Obesity Research. 2005;**13**(11):2021-2028

[55] Geerts CC, Grobbee DE, van der Ent CK, de Jong BM, van der Zalm MM, van Putte-Katier N, et al. Tobacco smoke exposure of pregnant mothers and blood pressure in their newborns: Results from the wheezing illnesses study Leidsche Rijn birth cohort. Hypertension. 2007;**50**(3):572-578

[56] Brion MJ, Leary SD, Lawlor DA, Smith GD, Ness AR. Modifiable maternal exposures and offspring blood pressure: A review of epidemiological studies of maternal age, diet, and smoking. Pediatric Research. 2008;**63**(6):593-598

[57] Brion MJ, Victora C, Matijasevich A, Horta B, Anselmi L, Steer C, et al. Maternal smoking and child psychological problems: Disentangling causal and noncausal effects. Pediatrics. 2010;**126**(1):e57-e65

[58] Kuciene R, Dulskiene V. Parental cigarette smoking and the risk of congenital heart septal defects. Medicina. 2010;**46**(9):635-641

[59] de Jonge LL, Harris HR, Rich-Edwards JW, Willett WC, Forman MR, Jaddoe VW, et al. Parental smoking in pregnancy and the risks of adult-onset hypertension. Hypertension. 2013;**61**(2):494-500

[60] El Marroun H, Schmidt MN, Franken IH, Jaddoe VW, Hofman A, van der Lugt A, et al. Prenatal tobacco exposure and brain morphology: A prospective study in young children. Neuropsychopharmacology: Official Publication of the American College of Neuropsychopharmacology. 2014;**39**(4):792-800

[61] Roza SJ, Verburg BO, Jaddoe VW, Hofman A, Mackenbach JP, Steegers EA, et al. Effects of maternal smoking in pregnancy on prenatal brain development. The Generation R Study. The European Journal of Neuroscience. 2007;**25**(3):611-617

[62] Huang CM, HL W, Huang SH, Chien LY, Guo JL. Transtheoretical model-based passive smoking prevention programme among pregnant women and mothers of young children. European Journal of Public Health. 2013;**23**(5):777-782

[63] Ohida T, Kaneita Y, Osaki Y, Harano S, Tanihata T, Takemura S, et al. Is passive smoking associated with sleep disturbance among pregnant women? Sleep. 2007;**30**(9):1155-1161

[64] Qiu J, He X, Cui H, Zhang C, Zhang H, Dang Y, et al. Passive smoking and preterm birth in urban China. American Journal of Epidemiology. 2014;**180**(1):94-102

[65] Knopik VS, Maccani MA, Francazio S, McGeary JE. The epigenetics of maternal cigarette smoking during pregnancy and effects on child development. Development and Psychopathology. 2012;**24**(4):1377-1390

[66] Suter M, Ma J, Harris A, Patterson L, Brown KA, Shope C, et al. Maternal tobacco use modestly alters correlated epigenome-wide placental DNA methylation and gene expression. Epigenetics. 2011;**6**(11):1284-1294

[67] Lee KW, Richmond R, Hu P, French L, Shin J, Bourdon C, et al. Prenatal exposure to maternal cigarette smoking and DNA methylation: Epigenome-wide association in a discovery sample of adolescents and replication in an independent cohort at birth through 17 years of age. Environmental Health Perspectives. 2015;**123**(2):193-199

[68] Levis DM, Stone-Wiggins B, O'Hegarty M, Tong VT, Polen KN, Cassell CH, et al. Women's perspectives on smoking and pregnancy and graphic warning labels. American Journal of Health Behavior. 2014;**38**(5):755-764

[69] Koren G. Nicotine replacement therapy during pregnancy. Canadian Family Physician Medecin de Famille Canadien. 2001;**47**:1971-1972

[70] Wehby GL, Wilcox A, Lie RT. The impact of cigarette quitting during pregnancy on other prenatal health behaviors. Review of Economics of the Household. 2013;**11**(2):211-233

[71] Cressman AM, Pupco A, Kim E, Koren G, Bozzo P. Smoking cessation therapy during pregnancy. Canadian Family Physician Medecin de Famille Canadien. 2012;**58**(5):525-527

Chapter 4

The Role of APC-Resistance for Predicting Venous Thrombosis and Pregnancy Complications in Carriers of Factor V Leiden (1691) G/A Mutation

Andrey Pavlovich Momot,
Maria Gennadevna Nikolaeva,
Valeriy Anatolevich Elykomov and
Ksenia Andreevna Momot

Additional information is available at the end of the chapter

http://dx.doi.org/10.5772/intechopen.72210

Abstract

This chapter presents the results of the prospective cohort study of 500 females with factor V Leiden, *FVL*, 1691 GA genotype, during 2008–2015. The association between FVL (regardless of its laboratory phenotype—factor Va resistance to activated protein C, APC resistance) and the development of VTEC (both outside of and during pregnancy) and gestational complications such as preeclampsia, fetal growth restriction, and miscarriage has been established. Additionally, the leading role of APC resistance degree in the clinical manifestation of *FVL* 1691 GA genotype as thrombotic events and pregnancy complications has been proved. Based on the data obtained, advanced approaches for the stratification of pregnant women into risk groups for the development of venous thromboembolic complications and pregnancy complications at different gestational ages adjusted for APC resistance degree are proposed. The found patterns can be useful in assessing the need for heparin prophylaxis during pregnancy from the standpoint of personalized medicine.

Keywords: APC resistance, factor V Leiden, thrombosis, preeclampsia, fetal growth restriction, miscarriage, ROC analysis

1. Introduction

In 1993, Swedish scientist Bern Dalbeck described hereditary thrombophilia that was caused by the inability of blood to react to activated protein C. A year later, in Leiden, Netherlands, Professor Roger Bertin managed to decipher the pathogenesis of this thrombophilia type.

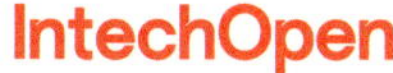

The pathology was called "factor V Leiden" [1, 2]. Factor V Leiden is a point mutation in the proaccelerin gene, accompanied by the substitution of the guanine nucleotide with adenine at position 1691 (*FV* G1691A), which leads to the substitution of the arginine (Arg = R) with the glutamine (Gln = Q) at position 506 (FV R506Q) in the protein chain that is the product of this gene. Due to this mutation, the resistance of factor V to the activated protein C (APC resistance) is formed [3]. This genetic deficiency is one of the most common causes of hereditary thrombophilia in European countries, and it is noted in 8–15% of the white population [4, 5].

Factor V Leiden carriage (a 1691G → A substitution) is traditionally considered as a genetic, non-modifiable risk factor for venous thromboembolic complications (VTEC) [6–8]. Moreover, the basis of risk stratification is the mutation genotype: the carriage of *FVL 1691 AA* is defined as a high risk; the carriage of *FVL* 1691 GA is defined as a moderate risk. VTEC in both carriage variants is most often associated with a precipitating factor, such as surgery, trauma, postpartum period, immobilization, hormone treatment or chemotherapy, or coexistence of other risk factors such as pregnancy, age, and comorbid conditions [7, 9–14]. The world community developed protocols and algorithms for the prevention of VTEC, depending on the degree of occurrence risk of the factor V Leiden mutation. However, the clinical manifestations of factor V Leiden are heterogeneous and can be not only in the form of thromboembolic events but also determine the risk of developing gestational complications, including the great obstetrical syndrome [15–17]. Modern ideas about the relation between *FVL* 1691 GA carriage and the risk of developing gestational complications are highly contradictory, the available studies in this direction are inadequate and ethnically heterogeneous and often contradict with each other [18–21]. According to the conclusions of world experts, it is impossible to make a final decision on the cause-effect relation between the *FVL* 1691 GA carriage and the unfavorable course of pregnancy.

Thus, it is not always possible to predict the likelihood of VTEC and obstetric complications with *FVL* 1691 GA carriage, based on the proposed and already proven risk factors. We believe that such risk depends not only and not so much on the factor V Leiden genotype but rather on its phenotype being an increase in APC resistance. However, in the existing recommendations for predicting the development of clinically significant events, the laboratory phenotype of the mutation—the APC resistance, whose magnitude actually determines the thrombosis tendency—is not taken into account.

The aim of this chapter is to outline the prospective approaches for stratifying pregnant women into risk groups for the VTEC development and for stratifying pregnancy complications based on the level of APC resistance, in order to address the issue of heparin prophylaxis during pregnancy from the standpoint of personalized medicine.

Materials and methods: Between 2008 and 2015, a prospective cohort observational study of 1100 Caucasian women was conducted, and 2707 pregnancy outcomes were analyzed in order to determine the clinical manifestation of *FVL* 1691 GA carriage in thrombotic events and gestational complications, such as preeclampsia, fetal growth restriction, and miscarriage.

The study was approved by the local research Ethics Committee of the Altai State Medical University (Protocol 5, from June 26, 2009).

Two cohorts were identified: the study group consisted of 500 patients with *FVL* 1691 GA genotype (mean age 30.2±4.7 years, the total number of completed pregnancies 1085), and the control group consisted of 600 women with *FVL* 1691 GG genotype (mean age 30.3±3.9 years, the total number of completed pregnancies 1622). Groups were comparable in age (p > 0.05).

Study group inclusion criteria:

- Female
- *FVL* 1691 GA carriage
- Age 18 to 45
- Informed consent

Control group inclusion criteria were the same as for the study group, but the patients were not carriers of *FVL* 1691 GA/AA.

Exclusion criteria:

- Age under 18 and over 45
- Autoimmune diseases, including antiphospholipid syndrome
- Chromosomal aberrations

In order to determine the relation between APC resistance with carriage of FVL and thrombotic events during pregnancy and gestational complications, within the framework of the study, APC resistance was diagnosed during pregnancy monitoring in 298 patients of the study group and 300 controls; the patients did not receive anticoagulants. To exclude the influence of confounding factors, which along with APC resistance expression can significantly affect the course and outcome of pregnancy, we defined additional inclusion/exclusion criteria for the groups.

Additional study group inclusion criteria:

- A singleton pregnancy that occurred in the natural cycle, confirmed by embryo viability at 5–6 weeks
- No abnormal development of internal genital organs
- No extragenital diseases in the stage of decompensation
- No anticoagulant therapy

Control group inclusion criteria were the same as for the study group, but the patients were not carriers of *FVL* 1691 GA/AA.

Exclusion criteria:

- Abnormal development of internal genital organs, multiple pregnancy
- Pregnancy, resulting from assisted reproductive technologies
- Extragenital diseases in the stage of decompensation

Eight points were chosen to assess APC resistance, taking into account the waves of trophoblast invasion and reflecting "critical" gestational ages: 7–8 weeks, 12–13 weeks, 18–19 weeks, 22–23 weeks, 27–28 weeks, 32–33 weeks, 36–37 weeks, and 2–3 days postpartum.

Preeclampsia was diagnosed according to the international consensus criteria: systolic blood pressure (SBP) ≥ 140 mm Hg and/or diastolic blood pressure (DBP) ≥ 90 mm Hg; in women with base hypotension, an increase in the SBP by 30 mm Hg and/or DBP by 15 mm Hg compared to the base values (arterial pressure in the I trimester of pregnancy), accompanied by proteinuria: daily protein loss of 0.3 g/l or more, any proteinuria recorded in a single urine portion [22]. Fetal growth retardation was defined as a condition with the fetal body weight and/or fetal abdomen circumference being below 10% for a given gestational age and/or the morphological maturity index lag of 2 or more weeks from the true gestational age [23].

APC resistance normalized ratio (NR) value was obtained with "factor V-PC-test" detection kit ("Technology-Standard" Ltd.).

Statistical data processing was carried out using MedCalc 14.8.1 statistical software package. The verification of the static series for normality was carried out using the Shapiro-Wilk's W-test. The laboratory data are presented as a median (Me), 95% confidence interval (95% CI), and interquartile range [25th and 75th percentiles]. Comparison of the series was performed using nonparametric methods (the Mann-Whitney U test). For the qualitative characteristic values, the absolute and the relative percentage values were given. The verification of statistical hypotheses on the coincidence of the observed and expected frequencies was carried out using the criterion $\chi2$ and Fisher's exact test. For binary characteristics, relative risk (RR) and 95% confidence interval (95% CI) were calculated. Maximum p value is <0.05. To determine the predictive value of the quantitative assessment of APC resistance in the development of pregnancy complications in the given points, the ROC curve was used, followed by the determination of the area under it (AUC). According to the literature, the AUC index exceeding 0.70 is clinically/prognostically significant. Accuracy (effectiveness, significance) of the test (Ac) was calculated as the percentage of the number of true diagnostic test results to the total number of results obtained:

$$Ac = \frac{TN + TP}{FN + TN + FP + TP} \times 100 \quad (1)$$

2. Clinical manifestation of *FVL* 1691 GA carriage in thrombotic events regardless of APC resistance value

According to experts of the Royal College of Obstetricians and Gynecologists [8], factor V Leiden is considered to be a constant risk factor for thrombosis in asymptomatic women. In our study, thrombotic events were registered in 70 (14.0% out of 500) women with *FVL* 1691 GA genotype versus 9 (1.5% out of 600) with *FVL 1691 GG* genotype, which has statistical significance [RR 9.3; 95%CI, 4.7–18.5; $p < 0.0001$]. In all nine cases in the control group, deep vein thrombosis (DVT) of the lower extremities was diagnosed. In six patients DVT was diagnosed outside of pregnancy and was caused in five cases by combined oral contraceptives (COC) (calf deep vein, four cases; iliac-femoral-popliteal segment, one case) in one case by locked intramedullary flexible osteosynthesis in the setting of diaphyseal tibial fracture (the second day of the postoperative period). In three cases, DVT was registered during pregnancy: one episode in the first trimester and two postpartum (the third and sixth days). In 70 *FVL* 1691 GA patients, 98 thrombotic events were registered in different periods of life: in 45 women (64.3% out of 70), a single episode of VTEC; in 22 (31.4% out of 70), 1 case of rethrombosis; and in 3 (4.3% out of 70) women, 2 cases of rethrombosis. We studied primary phlebothrombosis on the background of FVL 1691 GA mutation carriage (**Figure 1**).

The analysis showed that in 71.4% (50 out of 70) of cases, the primary thrombosis was the result of iatrogenesis (41 CHC and 9 surgical intervention). As it is known, administering estrogen-containing CHC is absolutely contraindicated for *FVL* 1691 GA patients [5, 24]; however, 63 patients of the study group were offered exactly this type of elective contraception that resulted in thrombotic events in 65.1% (41 out of 63) of cases. Thrombotic patients were administered medicines containing either 30 or 20 μg of ethinylestradiol. Out of 41 episodes of CHC-induced thrombosis, in 30 cases the process developed in the area of tibial veins and in 10 cases in the iliac-popliteal-femoral segment, and in 1 case, pulmonary embolism was diagnosed. During the treatment, two patients were implanted a vena cava filter.

Taking into account that estrogen-containing medicines are widely used in gynecology (contraception, menopausal hormone therapy, ovulation stimulation cycles, etc.), we calculated the risk of developing VTEC associated with CHC in *FVL* 1691 GA patients as 9.2 [RR 9.2; 95%CI, 3.9–21.9; $p < 0.0001$].

In 13 patients, *FVL* 1691 GA manifested itself as thrombosis after surgery, with 9 patients having the first episode of thrombosis and 4 cases with rethrombosis. All women underwent "small" surgeries, and according to the combined assessment of clinical data, they had a moderate risk of VTEC in the postoperative period [25], which implies prophylactic low-molecular-weight heparin (LMWH) administration according to the dosage regimen recommended by the manufacturer for moderate-risk patients [5]. However, none of the 13 patients received heparin prophylaxis. In 7 cases (10% out of 70), the primary thrombosis cause could not be established. All seven patients with idiopathic phlebothrombosis had an episode of

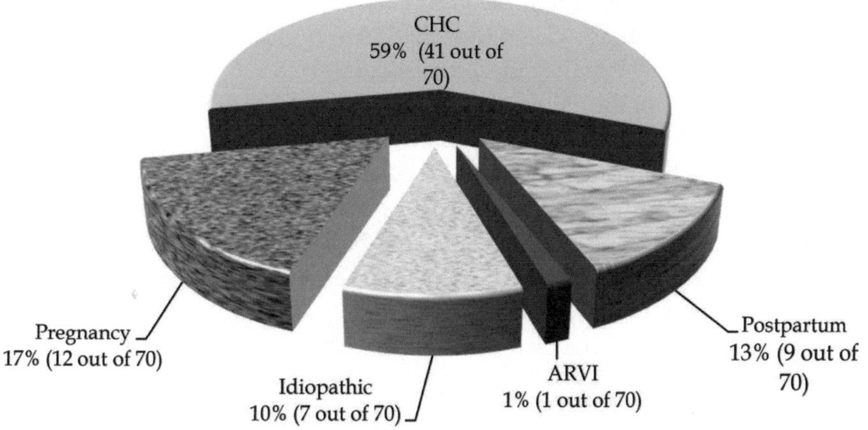

Figure 1. Primary phlebothrombosis proportion in *FVL* 1691 GA patients based on inducing factor. Abbreviations: CHC, combined hormonal contraceptives; ARVI, acute respiratory viral disease.

rethrombosis on the background of ARVI or after a surgical intervention within the first year. Viral infection, as a factor inducing primary thrombosis, was diagnosed in one case; three DVTs on the background of ARVI were recurrent.

In total, 65 thrombotic events occurred in 58 (11.6% out of 500) women outside of pregnancy; the frequency of rethrombosis was 12.1% (7 out of 65). During pregnancy, *FVL* 1691 GA was manifested in thrombotic events in 33 patients (6.6% out of 500), primary phlebothrombosis induced by pregnancy was registered in 12 patients (17.0% out of 70), and rethrombosis was registered in 21 cases.

For the convenience of perception, we identified groups of pregnant women according to the risk characteristics of VTEC development during pregnancy and postpartum given in clinical recommendations [8]:

1. Asymptomatic patients
2. A single episode of VTEC, associated with transient risk factors
3. A history with multiple episodes of VTEC

The number of pregnancies in asymptomatic *FVL* 1691 GA patients was 1027; in 58 cases thrombosis was registered before pregnancy. It should be noted that *FVL* 1691 GA genotype had not been considered as a risk factor for the development of VTEC during pregnancy and postpartum until 2015 [26]. Therefore, according to the clinical recommendations, these patients did not need antenatal VTEC prevention. In our study, the course of 12 pregnancies (1.2% of 1027) was complicated by an episode of primary VTEC, one case being vertebrobasilar basin thrombosis on the right, nine cases being tibial vein thrombosis, and two cases being iliac-femoral veins thrombosis.

According to the data obtained, we calculated the risk of *FVL* 1691 GA manifestation during pregnancy and postpartum in asymptomatic women compared to *FVL* 1691 GG patients. In our study, it is 4.7 [RR 4.7; 95%CI, 1.5–14.7; p = 0.0069].

Forty-five patients were included into the group with history of a single VTEC before pregnancy, whose thrombosis was associated with CHC or a surgical intervention. In 10 (22.2% out of 45) women, additional factors that affect the risk of developing VTEC were identified during pregnancy—a history of thrombosis in first-degree relatives up to 50 years, an implanted vena cava filter, and obesity (BMI, 25)—being the reason why they received prophylactic doses of LMWH throughout pregnancy and 6 weeks postpartum. With heparin prophylaxis, episodes of rethrombosis antenatally and/or postpartum were not registered. In 35 (77.8% out of 45) pregnant women with a history of thrombosis, the risk of VTEC was determined as intermediate, which presumed only postpartum LMWH prophylaxis for 6 weeks. In 18 (51.4% out of 35) patients who did not receive thromboprophylaxis, the course of pregnancy and postpartum were complicated by rethrombosis in the left lower extremity deep veins.

As known, patients with a history of multiple VTECs belong to the group with a very high risk of recurrent VTECs. In our study, this group includes 12 women: 6 of them had rethrombosis outside of pregnancy, and 6 had thrombosis in previous pregnancies. According to the

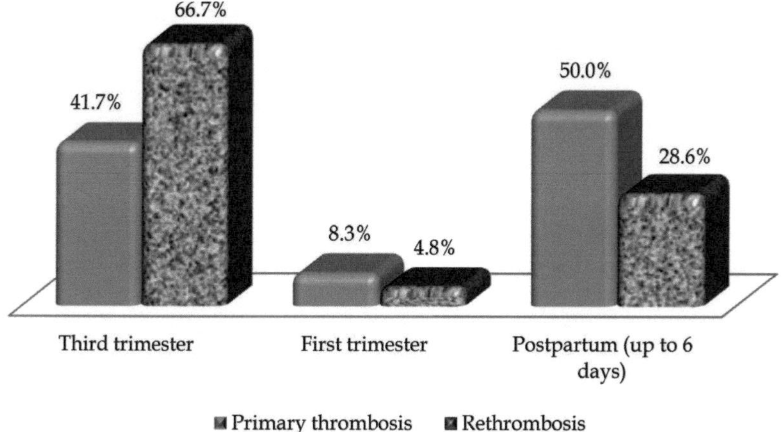

Figure 2. The periods of clinical manifestation of thrombotic events in *FVL* 1691 GA patients, depending on the personal thrombotic history.

available recommendations for VTEC prevention, patients of this group need antenatal and postpartum administration of LMWH. It should be noted that most patients did not follow the recommended continuous administration of LMWH. As a result, three (25.0% out of 12) pregnant women developed deep vein phlebothrombosis of the left lower extremity.

Interesting data were obtained during the analysis of the gestational age with a thrombotic event, depending on the personal history of thrombosis (**Figure 2**).

As can be seen, the major number of thromboses in our study was in the first trimester and postpartum. In the second trimester, thrombotic events were not registered. Perhaps this fact is due to mandatory thromboprophylaxis during the first 6 weeks after delivery in patients with a history of VTEC and without thromboprophylaxis in asymptomatic women [26].

3. Clinical manifestation of *FVL* 1691 GA in pregnancy complications regardless of changes in APC resistance

The question about the possible association between *FVL* 1691 GA and the risk of developing pregnancy complications remains controversial up to the present, despite the fact that one of the leading links in the pathogenesis of a whole range of obstetric complications is the imbalance between fibrinogenesis and fibrinolysis at the stage of trophoblast invasion, accompanied by microthrombus formation in placental vessels, by obstructive lesions of the myometrial segments of spiral arteries, and by abnormal placental perfusion.

Most of earlier studies, aimed at the chances of pregnancy complication development depending on the candidate gene and its genotype, were retrospective, ethnically heterogeneous, and sometimes not systematized. The peculiarity of our study lies in its prospective observational character and its seven-year period. Consequently, the course and outcome of 1085 pregnancies have been analyzed.

Upon completion of the study, an outcome analysis was conducted aimed at determining a possible association between *FVL* 1691 GA and its clinical manifestation in:

- Early reproductive loss (ERL)
- Preeclampsia (PE)
- Fetal growth restriction (FGR)
- Preterm birth (PB)

Early reproductive loss, as it is known, is a loss (an empty embryo sac or with an embryo) with a gestational age of up to 12 weeks [27].

The analysis of completed pregnancies showed 33.7% (366 out of 1085) of all pregnancies in *FVL* 1691 GA patients, and 10.3% (186 out of 1622) in patients with normal *FVL* 1691 GG genotype ended with early reproductive losses (ERL) [RR 3.0; 95%CI, 2.5–4.5; p < 0.0001].

In both groups, early reproductive losses in some patients were recurrent (**Figure 3**). The number of patients in the study group with two ERLs was 2.5 times greater than in the control group [RR 2.5; 95%CI, 1.7–3.7; p < 0.0001], and the number of patients with three or more ERLs, that is, those suffering from recurrent miscarriage, was 4.5 times greater in the *FVL* 1691 GA group [RR 4.5; 95%CI, 2.3–8.6; p < 0.0001].

We also determined the cause of reproductive losses in the groups (**Figure 4**). The proportions in spontaneous miscarriages and ectopic pregnancies were similar (p = 0.7643 and 0.24, respectively).

One in four pregnancies, 23.8% (258 out of 1085), with *FVL* 1691 GA ended as embryo death up to 12 weeks (70.5% of all ERL), which is nine times greater than with normal *FVL* 1691 GG genotype—2.6% (42 out of 1622) [RR 9.2; 95%CI, 6.8–12.6; p < 0.0001].

A more detailed analysis of non-developing pregnancies in *FVL* 1691 GA patients showed that in 65 cases (25.2% out of 258), pregnancy ceases to progress at a gestational age of 5–6 weeks, and in 193 cases (74.8% out of 258), pregnancy ceases to progress at a gestational age of 8–9 weeks, which contradicts previously obtained data stating that *FVL* 1691 GA is associated with embryo death at a gestational age of more than 14 weeks [12, 28, 29]. According to the histological investigation, anembryonic gestation was registered in 57 (22.1% out of 258) patients; in the remaining 201 (77.9% out of 258), embryo death was registered. Certainly, the knowledge of non-developing pregnancy etiology and histological evidence indicating the absence of an embryo favors a chromosomal abnormality of the embryo, but in our study, there was no karyotyping of the abortus, and therefore we cannot confirm or reject this hypothesis.

Thus, the data obtained indicate that *FVL* 1691 GA statistically significantly affects the cause and number of early reproductive losses. But, of course, this risk factor needs to be assessed in the context of additional predictors of reproductive ill-being in the individual.

http://dx.doi.org/10.5772/intechopen.72210

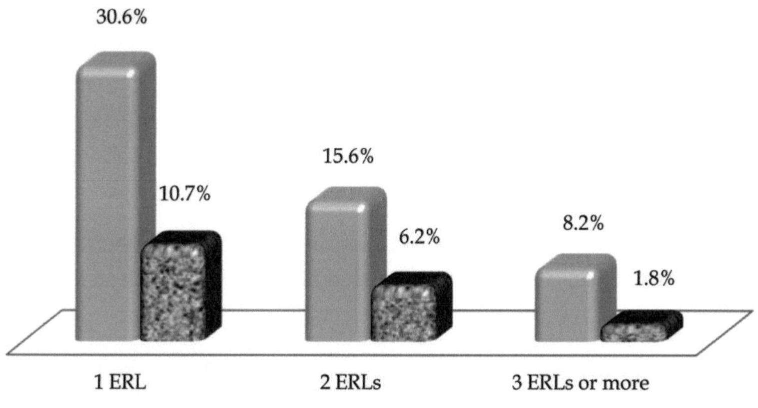

Figure 3. Proportion of women with one, two, and three or more early reproductive losses with *FVL* 1691 GA genotype and with normal *FVL* 1691 GG genotype.

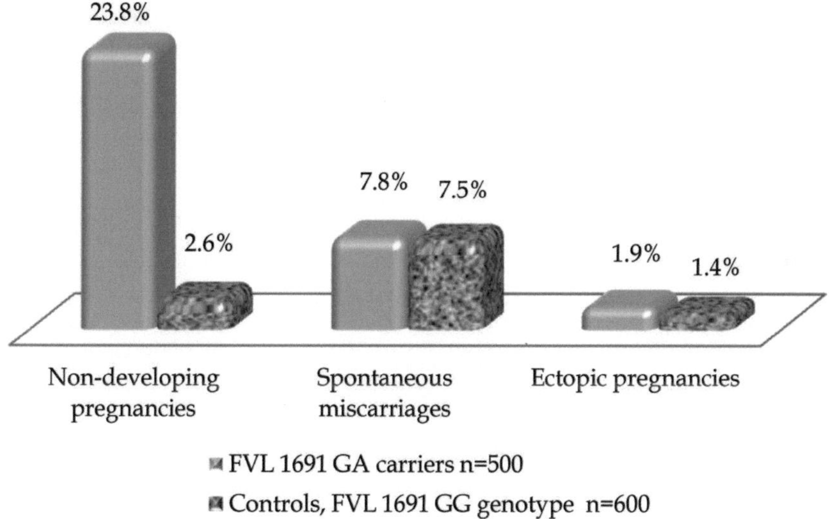

Figure 4. Proportion of ERL variants with *FVL* 1691 GA genotype and with normal *FVL* 1691 GG genotype.

Analysis of completed pregnancies in the *FVL* 1691 GA group showed that in 128 cases (11.8% out of 1085), pregnancy course was complicated by preeclampsia, which is statistically significantly greater than 52 episodes (2.9% out of 1622) with normal *FVL* 1691 GG genotype [RR 3.7; 95%CI, 2.7–5.0; $p < 0.0001$]. In this case, severe preeclampsia, as a pregnancy outcome, was registered in 28 cases (2.6% out of 1085) of the study group and in 8 cases (0.4% of 1622) of the control group [RR 5.2; 95%CI, 2.4–11.4; $p < 0.0001$].

In 130 cases (12.0% out of 1085), the course of pregnancy in the study group was complicated by FGR, which is statistically significantly greater than 64 episodes with normal *FVL* 1691 GG genotype (3.5% out of 1622) [RR 3.0; 95%CI, 2.3–4.1; $p < 0.0001$]. The weight of newborns with FGR in women of the study group was 1936.9±342.8 (95% CI 1805.9–2068.0); in the control group, it was 2124.9±274.2 (95% CI 1927.3–2321.5), thus having no statistical differences ($p = 0.1360$).

Given the pathogenesis unity of the placenta-mediated conditions, such as PE and FGR, we also analyzed the proportion of these complications in pregnancy outcomes in *FVL* 1691 GA patients.

In the study group in 33 (3.0% out of 1085) pregnancy outcomes, there was a combination of FGR and PE, versus 6 (0.3% of 1622) episodes in the control group [RR 8.2; 95%CI, 3.5–19.6; $p < 0.0001$]. In all six control group cases, the pregnancy was terminated prematurely (28–36 weeks) by an emergency abdominal birth due to life-threatening conditions of the woman and/or fetus. All six newborns were transferred to the second stage nursing; two children died during the first month of life.

With *FVL* 1691 GA genotype, the combination of FGR and PE in 7 (21.2% out of 33) resulted in antenatal fetal death (4 cases at 24–26 weeks, 3 cases at 28–30 weeks); preterm operative labor induction was performed in 27 cases (81.8% out of 33)—there were no intranatal and early perinatal losses.

Preterm birth is always considered to be an unfavorable perinatal outcome, whose degree depends not only on the gestational age but also on the causes: spontaneous or induced [30–33].

The proportion of preterm labor (PL) with *FVL* 1691 GA in our study was 7.1% (77 out of 1085), which is statistically significantly greater than 1.4% (26 of 1622) with *FVL* 1691 GG genotype [RR 4.2; 95%CI, 2.9–6.9; $p < 0.0001$]. The main PL difference is that PL before 28 weeks was only in the study group; 21 cases (27.3% out of 77) were registered. The number of PLs before 33 weeks of gestation was similar: 13 cases (16.9% out of 77) in the study group and 5 (19.2% out of 26) in the control group. There were 43 PLs (55.8% out of 77) in the study group and 21 PLs (80.8% of 26) in the control group with a gestational age of 34–36 weeks.

Structure analysis of PL is of interest. As is known, spontaneous PL is hard to manage, but it is well studied. Currently, prevention measures that have been developed and are widely used in practice are cervical incompetence correction, gestagen treatment, infection focus sanitation, and vaginal biocenosis normalization [34, 35]. PL due to medical reasons is always a catastrophe, being a condition that jeopardizes the life of a mother and/or fetus and thus ascertaining the need for early delivery regardless of the gestational age. As a rule, the main cause of indicated delivery is decompensation of placenta-dependent conditions.

In our study, the proportion of preterm labor induction with *FVL* 1691 GG genotype in our study was 26.9% (7 out of 26), which is consistent with general population data [31, 32] (**Figure 5**).

The proportion of preterm labor induction with *FVL* 1691 GA was 70.1% (54 out of 77), which is statistically significantly greater [RR 2.9; 95%CI, 1.5–5.5; $p = 0.0014$] than in the control group.

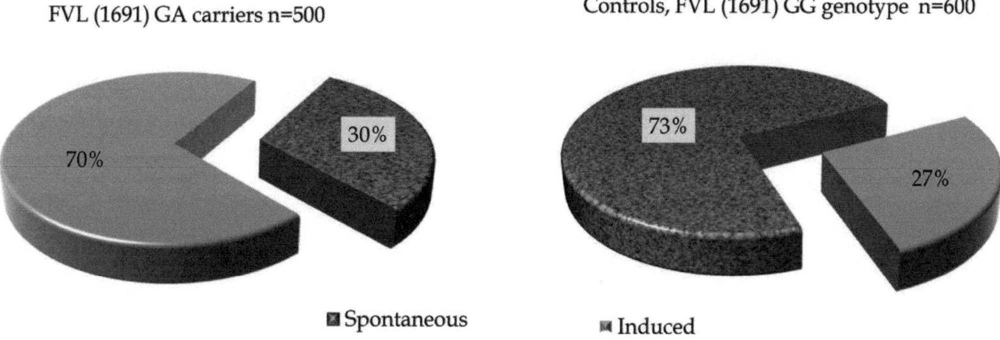

Figure 5. Preterm labor cause proportion in *FVL* 1691 GA carriers and controls.

Indications for induced PL with *FVL* 1691 GA genotype due to maternal condition were 8 cases with severe PE (10.4% out of 77) and 21 cases of placental abruption (PA) (27.3% out of 77). Due to fetal condition, there were 8 cases of progressive fetal hypoxia (10.4% out of 77) and 17 cases of antenatal fetal death (21.4% out of 77).

Summarizing the data presented above, we can note the following patterns:

1. The relative risk of developing VTEC outside of pregnancy in *FVL* 1691 GA patients is 9.3 [RR 9.3; 95%CI, 4.7–18.5; $p < 0.0001$]; when administering CHC it is 9.2 [RR 9.2; 95%CI, 3.9–21.9; $p < 0.0001$].

2. The risk of developing VTEC during pregnancy and postpartum in asymptomatic *FVL* 1691 GA patients compared to *FVL* 1691 GG patients is 4.7 [RR 4.7; 95%CI, 1.5–14.7; $p = 0.0069$].

3. *FVL* 1691 GA carriage is statistically significantly associated with early reproductive losses, increasing their number threefold [RR 3.0; 95%CI, 2.5–3.5; $p < 0.0001$], compared to normal *FVL* 1691 GG genotype.

4. With *FVL* 1691 GA, 70.5% of ERLs are non-developing pregnancies when embryo dies at 8–9 weeks, whose number is statistically significantly greater than with *FVL* 1691 GG genotype [RR 9.2; 95%CI, 6.8–12.6; $p < 0.0001$].

5. *FVL* 1691 GA is associated with the development of placenta-mediated conditions, increasing the risk of preeclampsia [RR 3.7; 95%CI, 2.7–4.0; $p < 0.0001$] and FGR [RR3.0; 95%CI, 2.3–4.1; $p < 0.0001$].

6. *FVL* 1691 GA is associated with a higher frequency of preterm birth, increasing their number 4.2-fold compared to normal *FVL* 1691 GG genotype [RR 4.2; 95%CI, 2.9–6.9; $p < 0.0001$].

7. With *FVL* 1691 GA, 70.1% of PLs are induced deliveries, which are statistically significantly greater than in patients with normal genotype [RR 2.8; 95%CI, 1.5–5.5; $p = 0.0014$].

A summary report on the clinical manifestation of *FVL* 1691 GA as thrombotic events and pregnancy complications is presented in **Table 1**.

Variable	Relative risk (RR)	95% confidence interval (95% CI)	P-value
VTEC outside of pregnancy in asymptomatic women	9.3	4.7–18.5	<0.0001
With CHC	9.2	3.9–21.9	<0.0001
VTEC during pregnancy in asymptomatic women	4.7	1.5–14.7	0.0069
Fetal growth restriction	3.0	2.3–41	<0.0001
Preeclampsia	3.7	2.7–4.0	<0.0001
Severe preeclampsia	5.2	2.4–11.4	<0.0001
Early reproductive losses	3.0	2.5–3.5	<0.0001
Non-developing pregnancy	9.2	6.8–12.6	<0.0001
Preterm labor	4.2	2.9–6.9	<0.0001
Induced labor	2.8	1.5–5.5	0.0014

A tabular report on the association of *FVL* 1691 GA with the risk of VTEC development and gestational complications.

Table 1. The relative risk of VTEC and pregnancy complications with ***FVL*** 1691 GA genotype.

The obtained data are consistent with the results of previously published meta-analyses and clinical recommendations [17–19, 21]. Nevertheless, despite an associative, statistically significant relation between *FVL* 1691 GA and the risk of VTEC development and pregnancy complications, up to now there are no international recommendations for the prevention of pregnancy complications in *FVL* 1691 GA patients. In order to determine a universal laboratory marker for possible ill-being, both thrombotic and gestational, we have attempted to examine the laboratory phenotype of the studied mutation as APC resistance, whose magnitude actually determines the tendency to thrombosis.

4. Relation between APC resistance in *FVL* 1691 AG patients and VTEC and pregnancy complications

The analysis of the NR, characterizing the degree of APC resistance, based on the genotype (*FVL* 1691 GA or *FVL* 1691 GG), showed that the APC resistance NR value median with normal genotype fluctuated at the study time points from 1.0 to 0.86 [95% CI 1.2–0.8]. At the same time, in pregnant women with *FVL* 1691 GA genotype, regardless of the pregnancy course, this value was significantly lower ($p < 0.0001$)—from 0.53 to 0.48 [95% CI 0.55–0.43] (**Table 2**).

According to the received data, the APC resistance NR value tends to decrease throughout pregnancy in both groups analyzed, regardless of the presence of a pathological allele. The nadir is at 28 weeks of gestation, when there is decrease of interstitial cytotrophoblast-invasive potencies, and gestational changes in the myometrial and endometrial segment of radial arteries of the uteroplacental area are completed. Further growth of placenta and fetus directly depends on the adequate remodeling of radial arteries and uteroplacental-fetal blood flow formation [10, 36].

http://dx.doi.org/10.5772/intechopen.72210

Group	Statistics	Control endpoints of the study							
		7–8 weeks	12–13 weeks	18–19 weeks	22–23 weeks	27–28 weeks	32–33 weeks	36–37 weeks	Postpartum
FVL 1691 GG	Me (95% CI)	1	0.95	0.9	0.88	0.86	0.86	0.88	0.9
		0.9–1.2	0.9–1.0	0.85–0.95	0.8–0.9	0.85–0.90	0.85–0.88	0.85–0.90	0.89–0.91
	25th–75th	0.9–1.05	0.9–1.0	0.85–1.0	0.8–0.95	0.83–0.90	0.8–0.90	0.8–0.95	0.8–0.91
FVL 1691 AG	Me (95% CI)	0.53	0.51	0.51	0.51	0.48	0.49	0.51	0.5
		0.52–0.55	0.50–0.53	0.50–0.53	0.44–0.51	0.43–0.51	0.48–0.50	0.5–0.52	0.48–0.51
	25th–75th	0.47–0.56	0.47–0.54	0.45–0.54	0.44–0.54	0.44–0.52	0.45–0.52	0.5–0.52	0.46–0.53
Mann-Whitney U		0	0	0	0	0	3	26	36
Test statistic Z		17.138	15.133	14.899	15.596	14.807	15.623	14.189	11.377
Two-tailed probability (p)		<0.0001	<0.0001	<0.0001	<0.0001	<0.0001	<0.0001	<0.0001	<0.0001

Table 2. APC resistance (NR value) depending on the presence of a pathological allele (***FVL*** 1691 AG or GG) in the groups at different gestational ages and 2–3 days postpartum.

With *FVL* 1691 GG genotype, the decrease in APC resistance NR value by 28 weeks in this study was 14.0% ($p < 0.0001$); with the heterozygous variant (*FVL* 1691 AG), it is 9.4% ($p < 0.0001$). Closer to the due date, there was an insignificant increase in the NR value: by 2.3% in the control group ($p = 0.1767$) and by 4.1% in *FVL* 1691 AG carriers ($p = 0.1265$) (**Figure 6**).

Here and below, the median is a marker; values corresponding to 95% confidence interval are the lower and upper vertical bars.

We conducted a study of APC resistance in 17 patients, whose pregnancy was complicated by vein thrombosis of the lower extremities. The NR value median showing the degree of APC resistance and preceding the episode of phlebothrombosis in the first trimester (7–8 weeks) was 0.49 [95%CI, 0.43–0.49]; in the third trimester (32 weeks), it was 0.48 [95%CI, 0.46–0.49]; 2–3 days postpartum, it was 0.44 [95%CI, 0.43–0.48], thus being statistically significantly lower than in the group with a normal pregnancy course (**Figure** 7).

Here and below, the median is a marker; values corresponding to 95% CI are the lower and upper vertical bars inside the "box"; the "box" is interquartile range between 25th and 75th percentiles; mustache is values corresponding to 2.5th and 97.5th percentiles; free elements are outliers.

At the next step, the APC resistance was analyzed depending on the course of pregnancy. In most cases in *FVL* 1691 GA patients with APC resistance between 0.58 and 0.5, pregnancy proceeded normally and ended with due date delivery. Moderate and severe PE were characterized by APC resistance between 0.48 and 0.43; with FGR the values were between 0.49 and 0.45. It should be noted that the increase in APC resistance in these outcomes was registered in 7–8 weeks of gestation already, when chorionic blood exchange develops and the first portions of uteroplacental artery blood enter the intervillous space [37, 38] (**Table 3**).

A more detailed analysis showed that the peak of APC resistance in the setting of FGR was at 18–19 weeks of gestation 6.2% ($p = 0.0239$); in the setting of PE, it was at 22–23 weeks 8.5% ($p < 0.0001$). In normal pregnancy course, the peak of APC resistance was at 28–29 weeks of gestation—8.9% ($p < 0.0001$) (**Figure 8**).

In order to predict placenta-mediated conditions with the APC resistance, we used the ROC analysis, which determined the threshold value of the predictor and the gestational age when the APC resistance has maximum chances to predict PE and FGR development. In this study, the following criteria for selecting the cutoff value have been defined: method sensitivity is ≥80%, the maximum total sensitivity and specificity of the diagnostic value. We also calculated the accuracy of the method (test effectiveness), which shows how many results were predicted correctly using this research method.

Table 4 summarizes the results of NR value ROC analysis assessing APC resistance at different time points as a predictor for the development of PE and FGR.

In accordance with the obtained results, we have determined the optimal cutoff for the APC resistance NR value in *FVL* 1691 AG patients for predicting PE and FGR, which was ≤0.49 for all studied gestational ages. The area under the ROC curve (AUC) at 8, 12, and 18 weeks of gestation proved high prognostic strength and clinical significance of this laboratory marker

http://dx.doi.org/10.5772/intechopen.72210

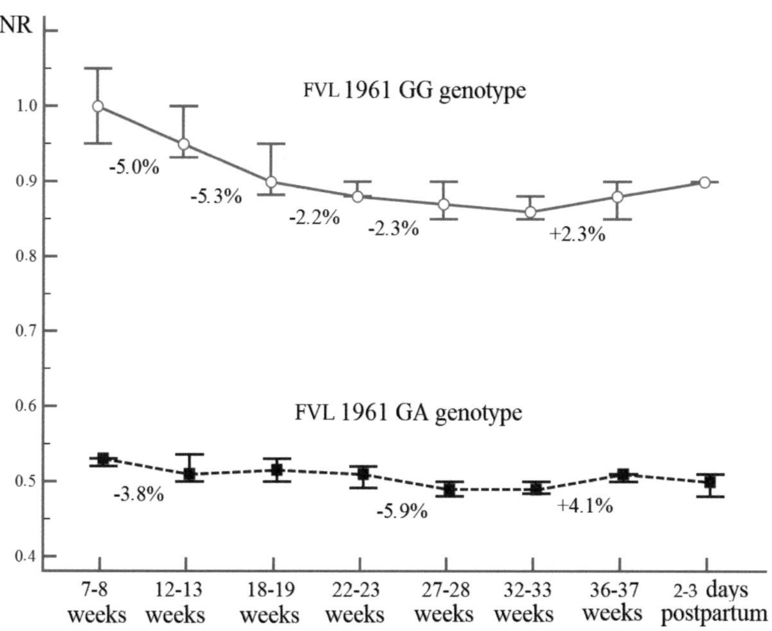

Figure 6. APC resistance depending on the presence of a pathological allele (*FVL* 1691 AG or GG) in the groups at different gestational ages and 2–3 days postpartum.

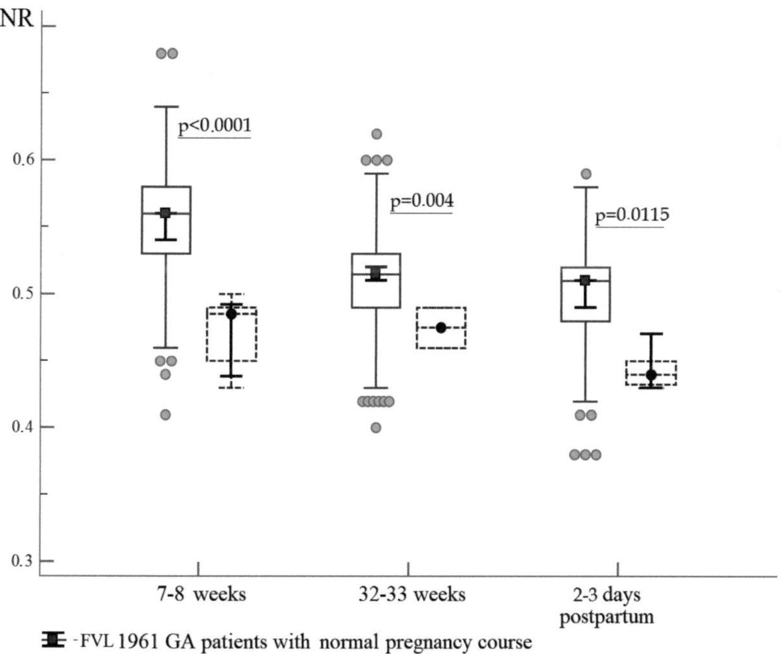

Figure 7. Values of APC resistance at the time points preceding thrombotic events in *FVL* 1691 GA patients.

Group	Statistics	Study points							
		7–8 weeks	**12–13 weeks**	**18–19 weeks**	**22–23 weeks**	**27–28 weeks**	**32–33 weeks**	**36–37 weeks**	**Postpartum**
NC n = 185 (1)	Me (95% CI)	0.56	0.54	0.54	0.53	0.51	0.51	0.51	0.51
		0.54–0.56	0.53–0.55	0.53–0.55	0.52–0.53	0.51–0.53	0.51–0.52	0.51–0.52	0.49–0.51
	25–75‰	0.53–0.58	0.51–0.58	0.52–0.55	0.51–0.54	0.50–0.53	0.50–0.53	0.50–0.52	0.48–0.52
PE n = 45 (2)	Me (95% CI)	0.47	0.45	0.45	0.43	0.43	0.44	0.49	0.51
		0.44–0.47	0.44–0.48	0.43–0.47	0.41–0.45	0.42–0.44	0.42–0.45	0.48–0.50	0.49–0.52
	25–75‰	0.44–0.48	0.43–0.48	0.43–0.48	0.41–0.45	0.41–0.45	0.41–0.46	0.47–0.50	0.48–0.52
FGR n = 58 (3)	Me (95% CI)	0.48	0.47	0.45	0.45	0.45	0.46	0.5	0.5
		0.47–0.48	0.46–0.48	0.43–0.46	0.44–0.45	0.42–0.46	0.45–0.47	0.48–0.50	0.49–0.51
	25–75‰	0.45–0.49	0.44–0.48	0.42–0.47	0.43–0.46	0.41–0.48	0.44–0.48	0.48–0.51	0.48–0.51
Mann-Whitney U (1/2)		925	254.5	328.5	267.5	95	436.5	748	473
Test statistic Z (1/2)		8.098	7.597	7.83	6.795	8.361	7.948	5.971	0.66
Two-tailed probability (p) (1/2)		<0.0001	<0.0001	<0.0001	<0.0001	<0.0001	<0.0001	0.0031	0.5096
Mann-Whitney U (1/3)		1267	493.5	506	556	248	957.5	1220	909.5
Test statistic Z (1/3)		8.778	8.552	8.492	8.057	8.677	7.052	5.267	0.545
Two-tailed probability (p) (1/3)		<0.0001	<0.0001	<0.0001	<0.0001	<0.0001	<0.0001	0.0611	0.5857

Abbreviations: NC, normal course; PE, preeclampsia; FGR, fetal growth restriction.

Table 3. APC resistance (NR value), depending on the course of pregnancy at different gestational ages and 2–3 days postpartum in ***FVL*** 1691 AG patients.

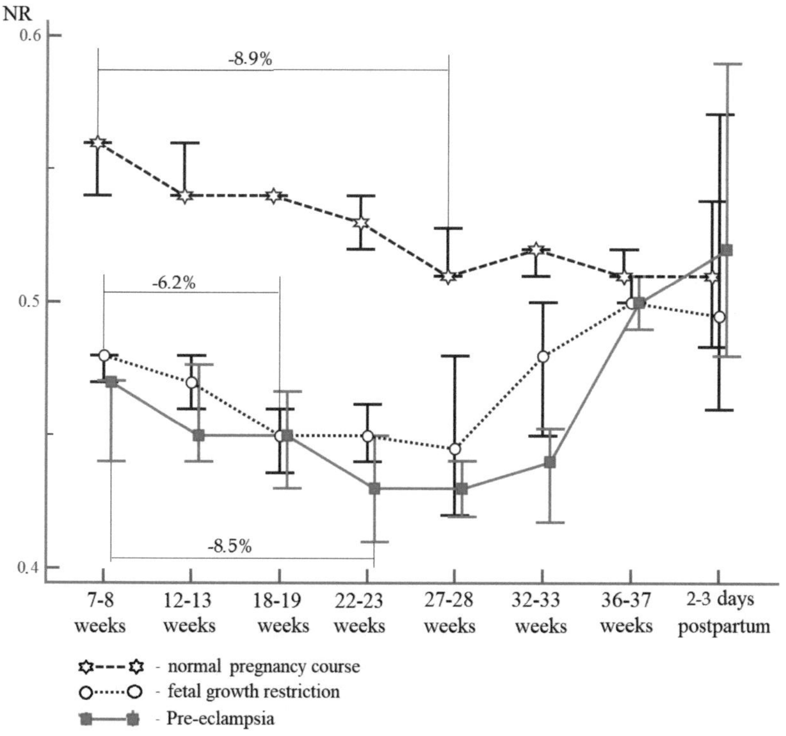

Figure 8. APC resistance in FVL (1691) GA patients with or without pregnancy complications.

for PE and FGR. The best AUC values (0.839 (95% CI [0.776–0.896], p < 0.0001) and 0.867 (95% CI [0.806–0.928], p < 0.0001) for PE and FGR, respectively) and the accuracy of the method (PE 86.2% and FGR 85.4%) were at 7–8 weeks (**Table 4**). ROC curves with maximum test effectiveness are shown in **Figure 9**.

In 25 *FVL* 1691 GA patients with embryo death before 12 weeks of gestation, APC resistance was also assessed. In all cases, the embryo death was registered at 8–9 weeks of gestation. NR median of APC resistance at 7–8 weeks of gestation in this group was 0.48 (95% CI, 0.41–0.49) and was statistically significantly lower than with further prolongation of pregnancy with a normal outcome—Me 0.56 (95% CI, 0.54–0.56, p < 0.0001) (**Figure 10**).

A critical disorder of uteroplacental area perfusion leads to decompensation of the placenta and, as a rule, is a reason for labor induction. We analyzed APC resistance in 29 women, whose pregnancy ended with indicated preterm birth. In 6 (20.7% out of 29) cases, preterm birth was due to decompensation of the intrauterine fetal condition, in 7 cases (24.1% out of 29), it was due to severe preeclampsia, and 16 (55.2% out of 29) cases were premature detachment of normally situated placenta.

Moreover, APC resistance at the time points before preterm birth was assessed, median NR of which had the lowest values (22–23 weeks 0.41 [95%CI, 0.40–0.43], 27–28 weeks, Me 0.42 [95%CI, 0.41–0.43]) in comparison with the same values at the studied time points with the development of PE and FGR (**Figure 11**).

Preeclampsia							
Statistical values	**8 weeks n = 45**	**12 weeks n = 45**	**18 weeks n = 45**	**22 weeks n = 45**	**28 weeks n = 43**	**32 weeks n = 40**	**37 weeks n = 38**
APC resistance NR value cutoff	≤0.49	≤0.48	≤0.49	≤0.48	≤0.48	≤0.49	≤0.49
Sensitivity	95.45	86.96	95.65	95.45	95.45	87.50	60.00
Specificity	66.38	69.64	66.02	68.93	66.31	64.91	66.67
The area under the ROC curve (AUC)	0.839	0.802	0.836	0.799	0.795	0.755	0.666
95% CI for AUC	0.767–0.896	0.716–0.900	0.764–0.907	0.749–0.830	0.738–0.831	0.679–0.815	0.530–0.802
P-value	<0.0001	<0.0001	<0.0001	<0.0001	<0.0001	<0.0001	0.0170
Accuracy of the test %	86.2	78.3	84.4	76.7	76.1	70.1	68.7
Fetal growth restriction							
Statistical values	8 weeks n = 58	12 weeks n = 58	18 weeks n = 58	22 weeks n = 57	28 weeks n = 56	32 weeks n = 52	37 weeks n = 49
APC resistance NR value cutoff	≤0.49	≤0.49	≤0.49	≤0.49	≤0.49	≤0.49	≤0.49
Sensitivity	96.77	97.06	96.67	85.29	90.00	93.33	61.06
Specificity	78.95	63.37	71.30	73.53	53.85	40.74	64.57
The area under the ROC curve (AUC)	0.867	0.815	0.805	0.766	0.769	0.679	0.651
95% CI for AUC	0.806–0.928	0.746–0.884	0.723–0.887	0.678–0.854	0.679–0.859	0.580–0.779	0.515–0.762
P-value	<0.0001	<0.0001	<0.0001	<0.0001	<0.0001	<0.0001	0.0180
Accuracy of the test %	85.4	78.6	82.7	79.2	72.3	64.2	63.1

Table 4. Results of ROC analysis in predicting PE and FGR at different gestational ages, using the APC resistance NR value in ***FVL*** 1691 AG patients as a marker.

The data we obtained, which indicate the relation between the APC resistance degree and the severity of the placenta-mediated conditions, bring us back to the second wave of cytotrophoblast invasion (18–28 weeks), whose quality depends on the completeness of myometrial radial arteries remodeling and intervillous space increase. Evidently, maternal coagulation disorder, which is also due to increased APC resistance, can lead to blood stasis, thrombosis on the

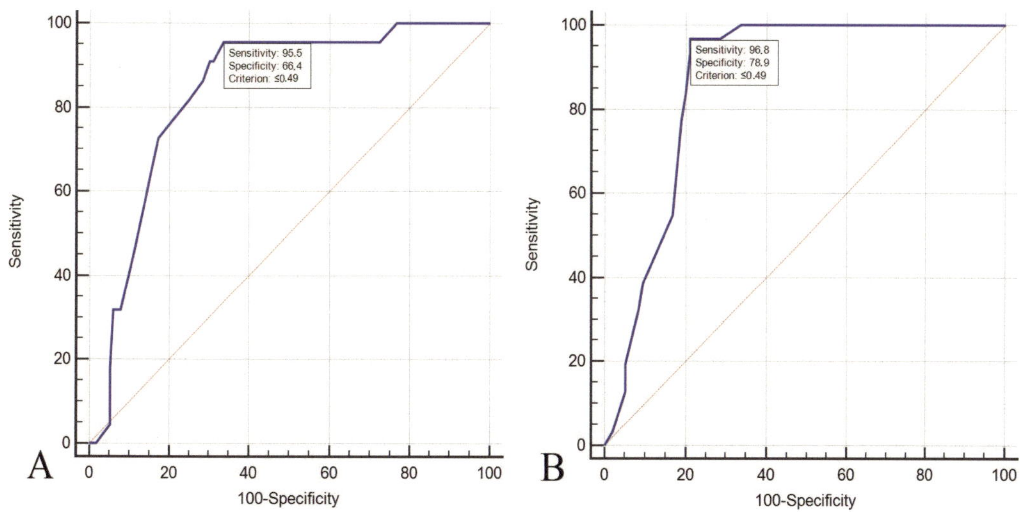

Figure 9. ROC curve for predicting the development of the placenta-mediated pregnancy complications based on the level of APC resistance in *FVL* 1691 GA patients. (A) The relation between APC resistance at 7–8 weeks of gestation and the development of PE. (B) The relation between APC resistance NR value at 7–8 weeks of gestation and the development of FGR.

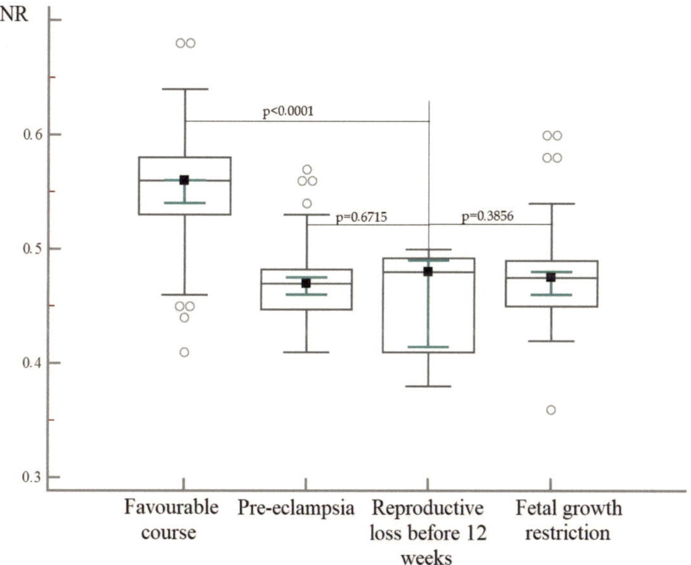

Figure 10. Median NR of APC resistance at 7–8 weeks of gestation in *FVL* 1691 GA patients depending on pregnancy outcomes.

surface of the syncytiotrophoblast microvilli, ischemia, damage, and invasive ability disorder. Clinically, this process can manifest itself either in ischemic placental disease [39] with FGR and PE or with the induction of microthrombosis from the area of destroyed microvilli and thrombosis increase in the intervillous space, followed by hematoma and placental abruption.

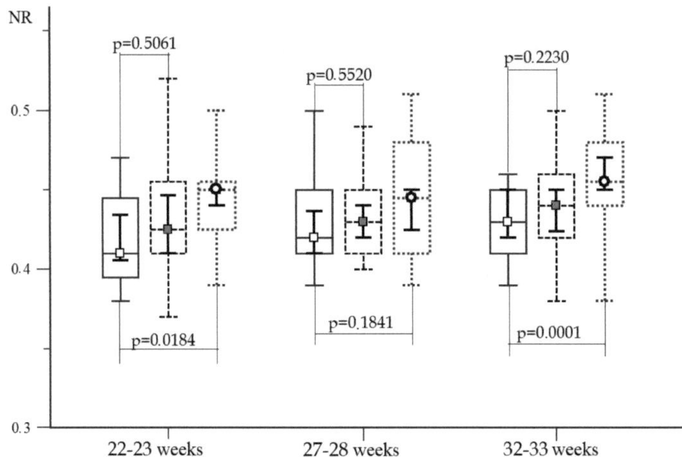

Figure 11. Values of APC resistance at gestational ages before the induced preterm birth in *FVL* 1691 GA patients.

Of course, APC resistance value cannot be considered the only and main factor of pathological processes. But its role in the development of placenta-mediated pregnancy complications is undeniable, which is confirmed by our study.

5. Conclusion

Heterogeneous carriage of FVL 1691 GA genotype, according to numerous studies, is associated with both thrombosis and pregnancy complications [17–19, 21, 40, 41]. In the study, *FVL* 1691 GA genotype clinical manifestation was close to that presented in the literature. In particular, outside of pregnancy the risk of developing VTEC increased 9.3-fold and 9.2-fold with CHC administration. At the same time, the risk of early reproductive losses increased 3-fold, 70.5% of which were missed abortions with embryo death at 8–9 weeks; the risk of developing preeclampsia increased 3.7-fold. There has been a 3-fold increase in the risk of fetal growth restriction, a 4.2-fold increase in preterm birth risk, and a 2.8-fold increase in indicated preterm delivery risk.

Despite the proven association of thrombosis and/or obstetric complications with FVL, the need for heparin prophylaxis remains questionable for such patients, as this mutation is not always clinically apparent. In our opinion, when making a decision on the use of anticoagulants during pregnancy, an additional criterion, APC resistance, can be considered, whose presence and degree, as are known, determine the tendency to thrombosis. We came to this conclusion after analyzing the frequency of clinically significant complications in pregnant women, with the normalized ratio values of APC resistance within the ranges of ≤0.49 to ≥0.50.

Thus, the presented data give grounds for considering the level of APC resistance as an objective laboratory criterion that allows not only stratifying patients into risk groups for thrombotic and pregnancy complications but also recommending antenatal heparin prophylaxis for FVL patients from the standpoint of personalized medicine.

Author details

Andrey Pavlovich Momot[1,2*], Maria Gennadevna Nikolaeva[1], Valeriy Anatolevich Elykomov[1] and Ksenia Andreevna Momot[1]

*Address all correspondence to: xyzan@yandex.ru

1 Federal State Budgetary Educational Institution of Higher Education "Altai State Medical University of Ministry of Healthcare of the Russian Federation, Barnaul, Russia

2 FSBI Altai Branch of "National Research Center for Hematology" of Ministry of Healthcare of the Russian Federation, Barnaul, Russia

References

[1] Bertina RM, Koeleman BP, Koster T, Rosendaal FR, Dirven RJ, de Ronde H, van der Velden PA, Reitsma PH. Mutation in blood coagulation factor V associated with resistance to activated protein C. Nature. 1994;**369**(6475):64-67. DOI: 10.1038/369064a0

[2] Dahlbäck B. The discovery of activated protein C resistance. Journal of Thrombosis and Haemostasis. 2003;**1**(1):3-9

[3] Dissanayake VH, Weerasekera LY, Gammulla CG, Jayasekara RW. Prevalence of genetic thrombophilic polymorphisms in the Sri Lankan population—Implications for association study design and clinical genetic testing services. Experimental and Molecular Pathology. 2009;**87**(2):159-162. DOI: 10.1016/j.yexmp.2009.07.002

[4] Heit JA. Thrombophilia: Clinical and laboratory assessment and management. In: Kitchens CS, Kessler CM, Konkle BA, editors. Consultative Hemostasis and Thrombosis. 3rd ed. Philadelphia: Elsevier Saunders; 2013. pp. 205-239. DOI: 10.1016/B978-1-4557-2296-9.00014-2

[5] Nicolaides AN, Fareed J, Kakkar AK, Comerota AJ, Goldhaber SZ, Hull R, Myers K, Samama M, Fletcher J, Kalodiki E, Bergqvist D, Bonnar J, Caprini JA, Carter C, Conard J, Eklof B, Elalamy I, Gerotziafas G, Geroulakos G, Giannoukas A, Greer I, Griffin M, Kakkos S, Lassen MR, Lowe GD, Markel A, Prandoni P, Raskob G, Spyropoulos AC, Turpie AG, Walenga JM, Warwick D. Prevention and treatment of venous thromboembolism. International consensus statement (guidelines according to scientific evidence). International Angiology. 2013;**32**(2):111-260

[6] Lockwood CJ, Krikun G, Rahman M, Caze R, Buchwalder L, Schatz F. The role of decidualization in regulating endometrial hemostasis during the menstrual cycle, gestation,

and in pathological states. Seminars in Thrombosis and Hemostasis. 2007;**33**(1):111-117. DOI: 10.1055/s-2006-958469

[7] Margaglione M, Grandone E. Population genetics of venous thromboembolism. A narrative review. Thrombosis and Haemostasis. 2011;**105**(2):221-231. DOI: 10.1160/TH10-08-0510

[8] Reducing the risk of venous thromboembolism during pregnancy and the puerperium. In: RCOG Green-top Guideline No. 37a. April 2015

[9] Baglin T, Luddington R, Brown K, Baglin C. Incidence of recurrent venous thromboembolism in relation to clinical and thrombophilic risk factors: Prospective cohort study. Lancet. 2003;**362**:523-526

[10] Gillet JL, Allaert FA, Perrin M. Superficial thrombophlebitis in non varicose veins of the lower limbs. A prospective analysis in 42 patients. Journal des Maladies Vasculaires. 2004 Dec;**29**(5):263-272

[11] Herrington DM, Vittinghoff E, Howard TD, Major DA, Owen J, Reboussin DM, et al. Factor V Leiden, hormone replacement therapy, and risk of venous thromboembolic events in women with coronary disease. Arteriosclerosis, Thrombosis, and Vascular Biology. 2002;**22**:1012-1017

[12] Robertson L, Wu O, Langhorne P, Twaddle S, Clark P, Lowe GD, et al. Thrombophilia in pregnancy: A systematic review. British Journal of Haematology. 2006;**132**:171-196

[13] Rossi E, Ciminello A, Za T, Betti S, Leone G, De Stefano V. In families with inherited thrombophilia the risk of venous thromboembolism is dependent on the clinical phenotype of the proband. Thrombosis and Haemostasis. 2011;**106**:646-654

[14] Wu O, Robertson L, Langhorne P, Twaddle S, Lowe GD, Clark P, et al. Oral contraceptives, hormone replacement therapy, thrombophilias and risk of venous thromboembolism: A systematic review. The thrombosis: Risk and economic assessment of thrombophilia screening (TREATS) study. Thrombosis and Haemostasis. 2005;**94**:17-25

[15] Momot A, Taranenko I, Tsyvkina L, Semenova N, Molchanova I. The risk factors of thrombogenic, thrombophilia, and the principle for heparin prophylaxis in personalized medicine. In: Özcan B, Murat B, editors. Anticoagulation Therapy. Croatia: InTech; 2016. pp. 47-67. DOI: 10.5772/61447

[16] Brosens I, Pijnenborg R, Vercruysse L, Romero R. The «great obstetrical syndromes» are associated with disorders of deep placentation. American Journal of Obstetrics and Gynecology. 2011;**204**(3):193-201. DOI: 10.1016/j.ajog.2010.08.009

[17] Wang X, Bai T, Liu S, Pan H, Wang B. Association between thrombophilia gene polymorphisms and preeclampsia: A meta-analysis. PLoS One. 2014;**9**(6):e100789. DOI: 10.1371/journal.pone.0100789. eCollection 2014

[18] Bates SM, Greer IA, Pabinger I, Sofaer S, Hirsh J. Venous thromboembolism, thrombophilia, antithrombotic therapy and pregnancy: American College of Chest Physicians Evidence-Based Clinical Practice Guidelines (8th edition). Chest. 2008;**133**(6 suppl):844-886. DOI: 10.1378/chest.08-0761

[19] Sergi C, Al Jishi T, Walker M. Factor V Leiden mutation in women with early recurrent pregnancy loss: A meta-analysis and systematic review of the causal association. Archives of Gynecology and Obstetrics. 2015;**291**(3):671-679. DOI: 10.1007/s00404-014-3443-x

[20] Rodger MA, Walker MC, Smith GN, Wells PS, Ramsay T, Langlois NJ, Carson N, Carrier M, Rennicks White R, Shachkina S, Wen SW. Is thrombophilia associated with placenta-mediated pregnancy complications? A prospective cohort study. Journal of Thrombosis and Haemostasis. 2014;**12**(4):469-478. DOI: 10.1111/jth.12509

[21] Ziakas PD, Poulou LS, Pavlou M, Zintzaras E. Thrombophilia and venous thromboembolism in pregnancy: A meta-analysis of genetic risk. European Journal of Obstetrics, Gynecology, and Reproductive Biology. 2015;**191**:106-111. DOI: 10.1016/j.ejogrb.2015.06.005

[22] Tranquilli AL. Introduction to ISSHP new classification of preeclampsia. Pregnancy Hypertension. 2013;**3**(2):58-59. DOI: 10.1016/j.preghy.2013.04.006

[23] Royal College of Obstetricians and Gynaecologists. The investigation and management of the small-for-gestational-age fetus. In: Green-Top Guideline No. 31. RCOG; 2013. [www.rcog.org.uk/en/guidelines-research-services/guidelines/gtg31/]

[24] Medical Eligibility Criteria for Contraceptive Use. 3rd ed. World Health Organization; 2004

[25] Caprini JA. Thrombotic Risk Assessment: A Hybrid Approach. Available from: http://www.venousdisease.com/J.A.Caprini-Hybrid Approach3-10-05.pdf

[26] Royal College of Obstetricians and Gynaecologists. Thromboembolic Disease in Pregnancy and the Puerperium: Acute Management. Green-top Guideline No. 28. London: RCOG; 2007. [www.rcog.org.uk/womens-health/clinicalguidance/thromboembolic-disease-pregnancy-andpuerperium-acute-management-gre]

[27] Farquharson RG, Jauniaux E, Exalto N, ESHRE Special Interest Group for Early Pregnancy (SIGEP). Updated and revised nomenclature for description of early pregnancy events. Human Reproduction. 2005;**20**(11):3008-3011. DOI: 10.1093/humrep/dei167

[28] Rey E, Kahn SR, David M, Shrier I. Thrombophilic disorders and fetal loss: A meta-analysis. The Lancet. 2003;**361**(9361):901-908. DOI: 10.1016/S0140-6736(03)12771-7

[29] Kist WJ, Janssen NG, Kalk JJ, Hague WM, Dekker GA, de Vries JI. Thrombophilias and adverse pregnancy outcome—A confounded problem. Thrombosis and Haemostasis. 2008;**99**(1):77-85. DOI: 10.1160/TH07-05-0373

[30] WHO. Recommended definitions, terminology and format for statistical tables related to the perinatal period and use of a new certificate for cause of perinatal deaths. Modifications recommended by FIGO as amended 14-10-1976. Acta Obstet Gynecol Scand. 1977;**56**:247-253

[31] Mercer BM, Goldenberg RL, Meis PJ, Moawad AH, Shellhaas C, Das A, Menard MK, Caritis SN, Thurnau GR, Dombrowski MP, Miodovnik M, Roberts JM, McNellis D. The preterm prediction study: Prediction of preterm premature rupture of membranes

through clinical findings and ancillary testing. The National Institute of Child Health and Human Development maternal-fetal medicine units network. American Journal of Obstetrics and Gynecology. 2000;**183**(3):738-745

[32] Ananth CV, Joseph KS, Oyelese Y, Demissie K, Vintzileos AM. Trends in preterm birth and perinatal mortality among singletons: United States, 1989 through 2000. Obstetrics and Gynecology. 2005;**10595**(Pt 1):1084-1091. DOI: 10.1097/01.AOG.0000158124.96300.c7

[33] Jackson RA, Gibson KA, YW W, Croughan MS. Perinatal outcomes in singletons following in vitro fertilization: A meta-analysis. Obstetrics and Gynecology. 2004;**103**(3):551-563. DOI: 10.1097/01.AOG.0000114989.84822.51

[34] Brown R, Gagnon R, Delisle MF, Maternal Fetal Medicine Committee. Cervical insufficiency and cervical cerclage. Journal of Obstetrics and Gynaecology Canada. 2013;**35**(12):1115-1127. DOI: 10.1016/S1701-2163(15)30764-7

[35] Flenady V, Hawley G, Stock OM, Kenyon S, Badawi N. Prophylactic antibiotics for inhibiting preterm labour with intact membranes. Cochrane Database of Syst Rev. 2013, 2013;**12**:CD000246. DOI: 10.1002/14651858.CD000246.pub2

[36] Urato AC, Norwitz ER. A guide towards pre-pregnancy management of defective implantation and placentation. Best Practice & Research. Clinical Obstetrics & Gynaecology. 2011;**25**(3):367-387. DOI: 10.1016/j.bpobgyn.2011.01.003

[37] Jauniaux E, Hempstock J, Greenwold N, Burton GJ. Trophoblastic oxidative stress in relation to temporal and regional differences in maternal placental blood flow in normal and abnormal early pregnancies. The American Journal of Pathology. 2003;**162**(1):115-125. DOI: 10.1016/S0002-9440(10)63803-5

[38] Mercé LT, Barco MJ, Boer K. Intervillous and uteroplacental circulation in normal early pregnancy: a confocal laser scanning microscopical study. Am J Obst Gynecol. 2009;**200**(3):315-320

[39] Ananth CV, Peltier MR, Chavez MR, Kirby RS, Getahun D, Vintzileos AM. Recurrence of ischemic placental disease. Obstetrics and Gynecology. 2007;**110**(1):128-133. DOI: 10.1097/01.AOG.0000266983.77458.71

[40] Sultan AA, West J, Tata LJ, Fleming KM, Nelson-Piercy C, Grainge MJ. Risk of first venous thromboembolism in and around pregnancy: A population-based cohort study. British Journal of Haematology. 2012;**156**(3):366-373. DOI: 10.1111/j.1365-2141.2011.08956.x

[41] Virkus RA, Løkkegaard EC, Bergholt T, Mogensen U, Langhoff-Roos J, Lidegaard Ø. Venous thromboembolism in pregnant and puerperal women in Denmark 1995-2005. A national cohort study. Thrombosis and Haemostasis. 2011;**106**(2):304-309. DOI: 10.1160/TH10-12-0823

Chapter 5

Respiratory Distress Syndrome Management in Delivery Room

Gianluca Lista, Georg M. Schmölzer and Ilia Bresesti

Additional information is available at the end of the chapter

http://dx.doi.org/10.5772/intechopen.73090

Abstract

The proper management of respiratory distress syndrome in the delivery room is a crucial step in the transition to extrauterine life, especially for preterm infants. In fact, it has been widely established that the optimization of the cardiovascular and the respiratory changes, which normally happen as soon as a term healthy baby is delivered, can have long-term effects. For this reason, every clinician approaching the delivery room should be aware of the consequences an inappropriate management could lead to and should know how to perform a proper resuscitation, using, where available, the most recent techniques. Regardless of the level of care provided by the hospital, there are some key interventions, which can be applied easily in every setting and are of crucial importance. In this chapter, we aim to provide a comprehensive overview of the most relevant measures to manage respiratory distress syndrome from the delivery room, starting from an explanation of the disease and moving toward the most recent evidence, from the basic concepts to the most advanced techniques to monitor fetal-neonatal transition.

Keywords: delivery room, respiratory distress syndrome, newborn, pathophysiology, gestational age

1. Introduction

The delivery room (DR) is the setting where the baby is given birth and where the neonatologist may have to assist the newly born infant in optimizing the transition from dependent fetal to independent neonatal life.

There is a wide consensus among clinicians about the importance of the DR management, especially regarding premature birth. In fact, the adequate management of unstable babies during the transition to extrauterine life can influence lifelong outcomes.

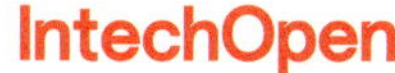

Providing optimal respiratory support is crucial to improve tissue oxygenation and guarantee normal gas exchanges. However, the physiological fetal-neonatal transition includes several crucial steps, which are difficult to achieve when the baby is extremely preterm. In fact, the lung and the chest wall of the preterm infants have essential characteristics making the newborn at the risk of developing respiratory distress syndrome (RDS).

1.1. Pathophysiology of RDS

The respiratory transition is usually recognized as a three-phase process, which reflects the three physiological status of the lung during the transition to extrauterine life.

In the first phase [1] of the respiratory transition, the lungs are fluid filled, and for this reason, no gas exchange can occur. Immediately after birth, with the first few deep breaths, a large tidal volume (V_T) is generated, followed by a cascade of physiological events, promoting the clearance of the fluid from the lungs and the establishment of pulmonary gas exchanges.

All these changes are critical for initiating postnatal circulation and for the achievement of an early and adequate functional residual capacity (FRC).

During the second phase, lung fluid should be prevented from re-entering the lung. In order to avoid the continuous opening and closing of the alveoli, endogenous surfactant and positive end-expiratory pressure (PEEP) play an important role in reducing surface tension and preventing alveoli collapse, respectively.

The third phase, then, is characterized by the initiation of gas exchange and the subsequent establishment of cardio-respiratory homeostasis.

While all these transitions are made by the healthy full-term newborn by himself within a few minutes after birth, preterm infants must deal with several physiological impairments to properly aerate the lung.

In fact, between the periods of viability (23 weeks' gestation) to 35 weeks' gestation, the preterm lung undergoes several complex anatomical and physiological changes, which include structural maturation, increase in surfactant production and storage, improved ability to clear fetal lung fluid, and enhanced epithelial barrier function. All these modifications progressively reduce the incidence of RDS, which falls to 5% when the baby is near term (> 36 weeks of GA).

RDS, also known as hyaline membrane disease, is the most frequent respiratory disorder in preterm infants. Over the last decades, the introduction of antenatal steroids and exogenous surfactant, besides significant improvements in ventilation strategies, have significantly improved survival rate, short-term complications, and long-term respiratory and neurodevelopmental outcomes of the preterm neonate.

RDS typically affects infants <35 weeks gestational age (GA) but older infants who have delayed lung maturation may be at risk as well. Low gestational age (GA) is the greatest risk factor for RDS (**Figure 1**), and its incidence varies inversely with birth weight among adequate for gestational age (AGA) infants (**Table 1**).

http://dx.doi.org/10.5772/intechopen.73090

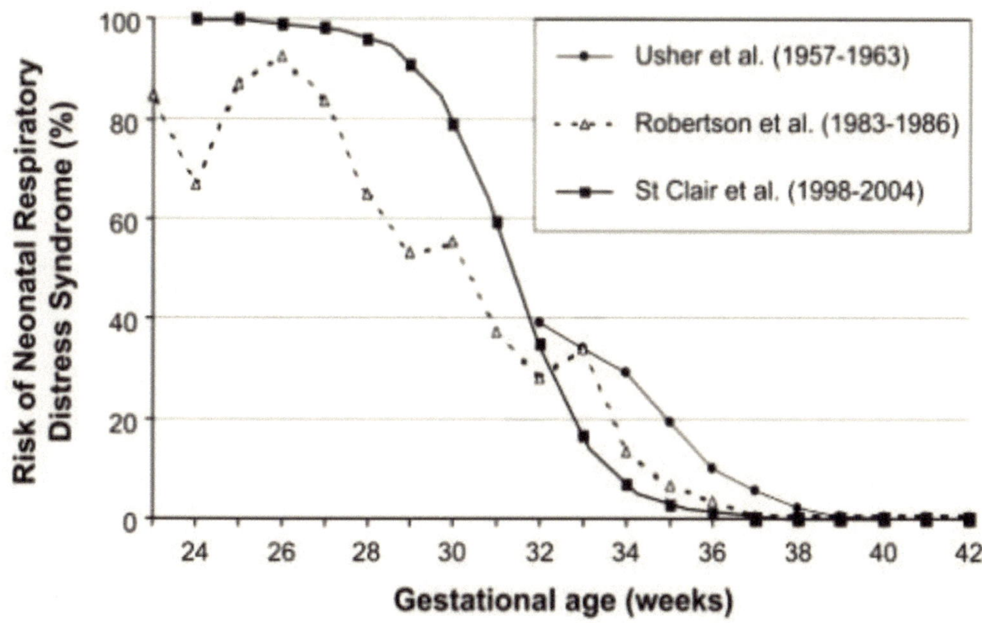

Figure 1. Risk of neonatal respiratory distress syndrome (RDS) as a function of gestational age and at different periods (current, from 1957–1963 prior to the introduction of antenatal steroids, and from 1983–1986 where ~40% of subjects received antenatal steroids). (da Caryn St. Clair "The Probability of Neonatal Respiratory Distress Syndrome as a Function of Gestational Age and Lecithin/Sphingomyelin Ratio", Am J Perinatol. 2008 September; 25(8): 473–480).

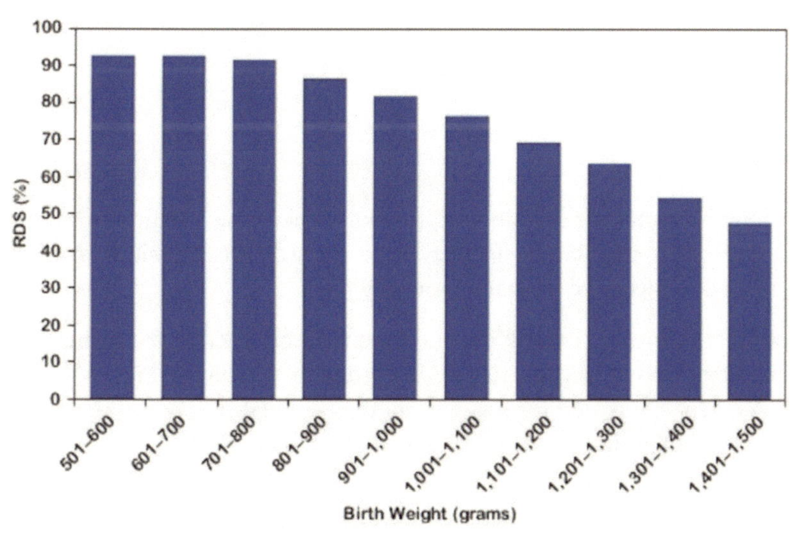

Table 1. Incidence of RDS by Birth Weight (BW) in the United States. Data from Vermont Oxford Network, 2003.

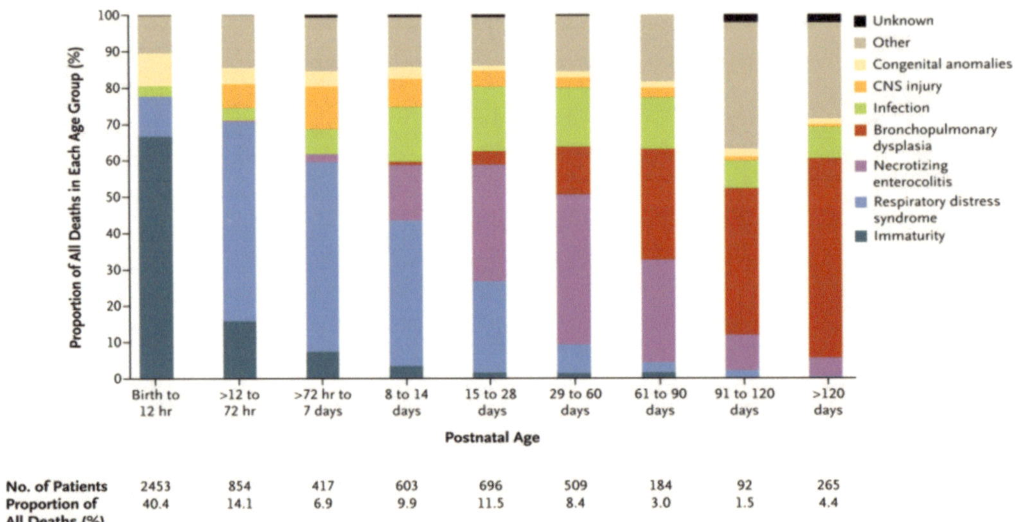

Figure 2. Proportionate mortality for major causes of death, According to postnatal age (da Ravi M. Patel et al, Causes and Timing of Death in Extremely Premature Infants from 2000 through 2011, N Engl J Med. 2015 January 22; 372(4): 331–340.).

The clinical diagnosis is made in preterm infants with respiratory difficulty, which includes tachypnoea, retractions of the rib bones, grunting respirations, nasal flaring, and increasing O_2 requirement. As shown in **Figure 2**, RDS plays a relevant role in premature infants' outcome in the first weeks of life, underlying how the proper ventilatory management is crucial for survival.

2. Interventions in the delivery room

2.1. Thermoregulation

Especially in preterm infants, maintenance of thermal homeostasis is crucial for the success of postnatal transition. This population, in fact, is particularly susceptible to cold stress and hypothermia, related to increased neonatal mortality [2–4].

Thermoregulation after birth is mainly dependent on the capacity of the neonate to activate thermogenesis using brown adipose tissue. Unfortunately, preterm infants lack sufficient brown fatty tissue deposition, and for this reason, they are highly exposed to an unequivocal tendency toward hypothermia once they leave maternal milieu.

The exact range within the newborn body temperature should be kept is not well defined, but using a target range of 36.5–37.5°C seems to be reasonable. On the contrary, mild neonatal hypothermia has been defined as mild when the body temperature is between 36.0 and 36.5°C, moderate at 32.0–35.9°C and severe below 32.0°C. There is a dose-related effect on mortality with an increased risk of approximately 30% for each degree below 36.5°C body temperature at admission.

Both hypothermia and hyperthermia should be avoided during stabilization and upon admission to the neonatal intensive care unit. Of note, low temperature worsens the susceptibility of premature infants to hypoglycemia. Cold stress with following altered pulmonary vascular tone and metabolic acidosis can worsen respiratory transition and trigger respiratory failure onset.

Systematic monitoring of temperature during resuscitation (preferably skin and rectal) is therefore mandatory to prevent inappropriate uncontrolled temperature variations.

Strategies to minimize heat loss include occlusive wrapping, exothermic warming mattress, warmed humidified resuscitation gases, polyethylene caps, and adequate DR temperature.

It is recommended that DR should be maintained at a temperature ranging 23–26°C, to the upper limits when expecting the birth of a very preterm infant (<28 weeks' gestation) [5]. Then, all infants below 28 weeks' gestation or <1500 g should be wrapped in polyethylene or polyurethane bags [6] up to their necks as soon as they are delivered, without being previously dried, to reduce heat loss and keep an adequate humidity [7]. The head coverage is fundamental, regardless of the material used for the hats, for two main reasons: the brain is a primary heat-producing organ and the head represents an extensive component of the neonatal body surface area.

Exothermic mattresses and radiant heaters are also recommended, with an accurate control of the babies' temperature especially after the first 10 minutes after birth, when the risk of hyperthermia substantially increases [5, 8].

An attractive way to promote thermoregulation is the application of skin-to-skin contact as a means of preventing heat loss at birth. This alternative is obviously applicable only to infants requiring minimal stabilization at delivery, assuming that techniques of skin-to-skin contact are carefully performed.

2.2. Ventilatory strategies promoting airway liquid clearance and alveolar recruitment

As previously mentioned, the preterm neonate, particularly that of an extremely low gestational age (ELGAN), often has limitations in achieving and maintaining "adequate" lung volume, mainly because surfactant production and storage are not sufficient and the respiratory effort is not effective [9].

In a preterm infant, lung volume optimization from the first breath should lead to a more physiological transition to neonatal life while maintaining adequate gas exchange and preventing, or at least limiting, lung injury [10].

The achievement of an adequate FRC at birth seems to be a crucial point for noninvasive respiratory support success.

To facilitate this achievement, reduced lung damage and improved oxygenation, continuous positive airway pressure (CPAP) has been advocated as the optimal strategy for the initiation of respiratory support [11–13]. If an infant fails to breathe spontaneously, current neonatal resuscitation guidelines recommend positive pressure ventilation (PPV) via a face mask [14].

Devices through which PPV can be applied are different according to the level of care provided by the unit.

Ventilation bags are the most easily found in the delivery room, and given the small V_T of neonates (4–8 mL/kg), they should not be larger than 750 ml to avoid excessive volume delivery and therefore volutrauma.

There are two types of ventilation bags: self-inflating bags and flow-inflating bags. The first one is relatively easier to use, and the recoil of the bags allows refilling even with no compressed gas source. Most self-inflating bags have a pressure release valve to prevent excessive pressure build-up and should release at approximately 30–35 cmH_2O. To deliver 100% oxygen, the bags must be connected to an oxygen reservoir. Otherwise, a maximum of 40% oxygen will be reached.

The flow-inflating bag only inflates when compressed gas is flowing into it, and the patient outlet is occluded. Proper use of flow-inflating bag requires a relative more training and practice.

Neither of these devices is optimal for the stabilization of preterm infants needing CPAP, because self-inflating bags cannot deliver positive pressure continuously, and on the other hand appropriate levels of CPAP are difficult to achieve and maintain with a flow-inflating bag. The T-piece resuscitator is the most widespread device in neonatal units, and like the flow-inflating bag, depends upon a compressed gas source and requires a tight face mask or endotracheal tube to inflate the lungs. With T-piece, it is easier to set and maintain PEEP and to administer PPV. One example of a T-piece resuscitator is the Neopuff™, which is flow-controlled and pressure-limited and specifically designed for application in neonatal settings. There is no wide consensus about which is the optimal PEEP to start resuscitation with. However, the latest ERC guidelines suggest a value around 5–6 cmH_2O [14], while the European Consensus recommends at least 6 cmH_2O to be individualized according to clinical condition, oxygenation, and perfusion [8].

Recent studies on preterm lamb have shown that a stepwise PEEP strategy at birth emphasizing time- and pressure-based recruitment and titrated to the subject's lung mechanics was feasible and demonstrated short-term beneficial results [15]. An observational study describing DR management with stepwise increments of PEEP (e.g., from 8 to 14 cmH_2O) plus surfactant administration among infants <26 weeks GA was shown to improve the rates of survival and morbidity, and reduce the need for mechanical ventilation (MV) [16]. However, since this approach included other interventions that may have interfere the final outcomes, there is a need for further evidence from a randomized trial before gaining wide acceptance.

There are several situations in which using bag and mask or a T-piece resuscitator is not sufficient to provide an efficient ventilation, which is the most important goal to achieve to guarantee normal perfusion and therefore normal gas exchange. The most likely cause for heart rate (HR) < 60 bpm, in fact, is deficient oxygenation of the cardiac tissue.

http://dx.doi.org/10.5772/intechopen.73090

Tube size (internal diameter)	Birth weight (g)	Gestational age (weeks)
2.5	<1000	<26
3	1000–2000	27–34
3.5	2000–3000	35–40
3.5–4	>3000	>38

Table 2. Suggestions for ETT size (Wyllie P, Neonatal Endotracheal Intubation, Arch Dis Child Educ Pract Ed. 2008 Apr; 93(2):44-9).

When ventilation with these devices does not show effects on chest expansion, HR and/or saturation of peripheral oxygen (SpO_2) or when PPV mask ventilation is prolonged, endotracheal intubation must be considered.

Supplies and equipment for endotracheal intubation should be readily available in the DR.

Intubation can be performed orally or nasally, although the oral way is usually preferred in emergency intubation because it is faster and easier to perform. However, both these techniques have their unique complications and share a few as well.

The tube size should be usually chosen according to the estimated weight of the newborn and/or to gestational age. Suggestions are shown in **Table 2**. However, other clinical considerations must be taken into account (e.g., nares size, malformations, glottis dimension, etc.).

To properly insert the tube at the right depth, a practical rule can be used:

Weight of the baby (kg) + 6 = position of the tube (cm); for example, 2 (kg) + 6 = 8 cm

Another popular way to rapidly calculate the depth of the endotracheal tube insertion is the "7-8-9 rule," which is translated into a baby weighing 1 kg intubated to 7 cm, an infant of 2 kg to 8 cm and one of 3 kg to 9 cm. This method should not be applied in neonates < 750 g [17].

After having achieved alveolar recruitment in the DR, with the initiation of gas exchanges and clearance of lung fluid, is of great importance to maintain a constant distending pressure in the airway using CPAP or PPV, to avoid losing the acquired FRC. For this reason, transport to the neonatal unit must be done with extreme care and should aim at guaranteeing a reliable administration of pressure in the recently recruited lung, always trying to limit the risk of lung injury.

2.3. Heart rate and oxygen saturation

During resuscitation maneuvers, HR and SpO_2 are monitored continuously using pulse oximetry, because they reflect the efficacy of the fetal-neonatal transition process [5].

The pulse oximeter should be placed on the right hand or wrist of the infant as soon as the baby is placed on the resuscitation trolley.

During neonatal resuscitation, an increase in HR is an indicator for effective ventilation [5, 18].

For this reason, a quick and reliable detection of the cardio-respiratory parameters is crucial to optimize critical interventions [19]. In fact, it has been demonstrated that alternative methods such as evaluation of HR using the stethoscope or palpation of the umbilical cord are not as accurate, especially in extremely preterm infants and when the baby is bradycardic [20–23].

Recently, besides the use of pulse oximetry, ECG monitoring has been proposed as an alternative to display HR during resuscitation [24]. However, challenging ECG lead placement on the wet skin, epidermal loss at the site of leads placement, and overestimation of HR in the setting of potential pulseless electric activity need a particular skill by the clinician to avoid delay in resuscitation maneuver.

Since in utero, the fetus is exposed to low relative blood oxygen tension, and thus fetal life occurs in a hypoxic environment, defining specific ranges for normal HR and SpO_2 at birth has been a priority for a rational use of oxygen therapy in the DR.

Preterm infants, in fact, are at high risk for hyperoxia-induced damages due to the immaturity of the mechanism that protects against oxygen free radicals. For this reason, avoid inappropriate O_2 administration, and consequently useless interventions, are mandatory. With the aim of correctly titrating fraction of inspired oxygen (FiO_2) in the DR, Dawson et al. have defined the range values for SpO_2 and HR in the newly born infants, which are now incorporated into resuscitation guidelines (**Figure 3**).

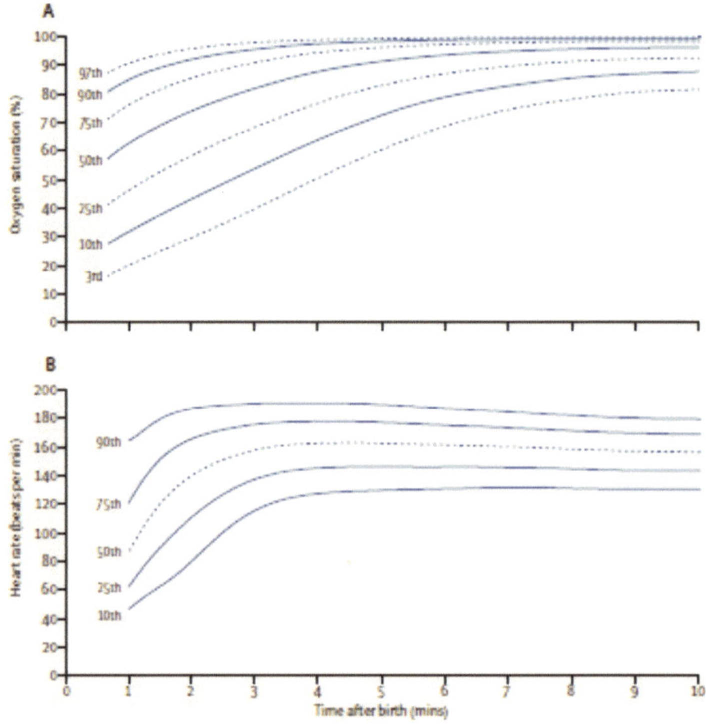

Figure 3. Normal ranges of heart rate and SpO_2 within the first 10 min of life in term and preterm infants who received no medical intervention at birth (Dawson et al.).

However, there is currently uncertainty about the optimal oxygen concentration at which starting resuscitation of preterm infants.

Considering what is shown in a meta-analysis by Saugstad et al. [25], resuscitation of term infants in air reduced mortality in comparison with resuscitation with 100% oxygen. Thus, babies born at term and near-term should initially be resuscitated with air (FiO_2 21%). On the other hand, very preterm infants who are initially resuscitated with air nearly always receive some supplemental oxygen in the subsequent minutes [18, 26]. Then, it seems that starting with intermediate FiO_2 titrating in the course of resuscitation is more appropriate for very preterm infants. Pending further evidence, the latest International guidelines on resuscitation [5] now strongly recommend initiating stabilization of preterm infants less than 35 weeks gestation with lower initial FiO_2 (21–30%). They also advocate against using high oxygen concentrations (65–100%), underlying instead the importance of not exposing these infants to additional oxygen without proven benefit.

2.4. Sustained inflation

Sustained inflation (SI) is defined as "a positive pressure inflation designed to establish FRC and applied over a longer period of time than would normally be used to deliver subsequent tidal inflations" [27].

The rationale behind SI relies on the concept that maintaining positive pressure for a prolonged time provides the lung with the necessary pressure gradient to drive the fluid along the airways distally and aiding transition in infants with inadequate respiratory effort.

For this reason, the SI maneuver is an intriguing approach to allow premature infants to achieve an FRC rapidly. This experimental maneuver has been successfully used to recruit the lung in the early transitional phase to extrauterine life and in preventing repeated collapse and the opening of alveoli preterm animal models [28]. Reports of prompt increases in HR, as well as cerebral and systemic oxygenation in preterm infants exposed to SI in the DR, are signs suggestive of a positive effect of this maneuver [29].

Studying the resuscitation of asphyxiated near-term infants, Vyas et al [30] observed that the first inflations considered at the end of a 1" inflation gas were still entering the lung. Hence, they speculated that a longer inflation time would increase the Vt. They showed that in maintaining the initial inflation for approximately 5", the Vt was doubled. According to these findings, the latest ERC neonatal guidelines recommend to maintain the initial pressure for 2–3" for the first five inflations [14].

Sustained inflation can be delivered with a face mask or through an endotracheal tube. However, effects on infants [31, 32] using face masks have shown to be less impressive than using a tube in animal models [33], probably because of the tendency toward active closure of the glottis in infants during apnea or hypoxia [34, 35].

Observational studies analyzing the effect of SI in the have reported a significant reduction in rates of intubation and MV, bronchopulmonary dysplasia (BPD), and use of oxygen [36], which led to the design of several randomized controlled trials to compare SI with PPV alone [31, 37].

However, there is a lack of data regarding the optimal pressure to deliver and the best duration of the prolonged inflation. Thus, concerns regarding the safety of this technique still need to be clarified. A potential method could be end-tidal CO_2 ($ETCO_2$) monitoring, which have shown to be feasible to guide length of SI during resuscitation [38]. Also, the effectiveness of SI maneuver can be largely influenced by several factors, such as the different skill of the clinical team, interface through which a SI is delivered [39], the infant's respiratory effort [35] and mask leak [32]. Given these findings, SI might not be the optimal approach in all apneic infants.

This data, besides the paucity of large well-designed RCT on the routine use of SI, especially in the most premature infants, suggest that its application should be actually limited to research settings, in according with AAP [40] and ERC guidelines [14].

2.5. Surfactant administration

The introduction of surfactant replacement therapy in early 1990s was a milestone in the treatment of preterm babies, leading to a significant reduction in mortality and to a different approach in respiratory problems of premature neonates. In fact, exogenous surfactant is nowadays routinely used in clinical practice to treat RDS.

The types of surfactant currently commercialized are animal-derived and are obtained from either bovine or porcine lungs.

Due to its composition, surfactant can reduce surface tension on the inner surface of the alveoli, thus preventing alveoli from collapsing during expiration.

In the last decades, the use of surfactant has changed consistently, and recommendations for its administration have been modified. For decades, the standard stabilization method for very preterm infants <29 weeks GA was endotracheal intubation and surfactant replacement therapy in the DR. However, a recent Cochrane meta-analysis [41] concluded that thanks to the widespread use of antenatal steroids and noninvasive respiratory support, routine prophylactic surfactant treatment provides no advantage over selective surfactant administration. In fact, prophylactic intubation and surfactant administration, compared with early noninvasive CPAP therapy, does not reduce BPD risk in preterm infants [12, 42, 43].

However, the efficacy of noninvasive respiratory support is closely related to GA. Among very low birth weight (VLBW) infants initially managed with N-CPAP about 50% of needs subsequent intubation and MV [11]. For this reason, in very preterm infants, *early rescue* surfactant therapy seems to be appropriate [36, 44] and should be considered early in the DR or immediately at NICU entry. According to the latest Consensus on the management of RDS [8], babies showing signs of RDS are recommended to be treated with early surfactant rescue therapy, and if the baby needs intubation surfactant should be given.

Providing early rescue surfactant (within the first 2 h of life) to mechanically ventilated preterm infants, as compared with delayed surfactant administration (after the second hour of life), reduces the risk of BPD and the composite of death or BPD (RR 0.83, 95% CI 0.75–0.91) [45].

As mentioned previously, prenatal history must be carefully considered among the criteria for surfactant administration (especially prenatal steroids which promotes lungs' maturation).

As it is noted from literature MV, especially when prolonged, has been widely shown to be associated with BPD onset, neurodevelopmental impairment and death [12, 46]. With the aim to reduce these risks, limiting endotracheal ventilation, the so-called INSURE procedure was introduced in clinical practice. It combines intubation, surfactant treatment, then rapid extubation back to noninvasive respiratory support.

Recently, other strategies to administer surfactant avoiding endotracheal intubation and subsequent MV are gaining in popularity [47–49]. They are commonly called "LISA" (Less Invasive Surfactant Administration) or "MIST" (Minimally Invasive Surfactant Therapy). Kribs et al. perform direct laryngoscopy and using a Magill forceps place a feeding tube in the trachea, with no premedication [50, 51]. Overall, the need for MV was reduced; however, no differences in BPD or death were observed. [47]

The MIST technique uses a narrow-bore tracheal catheter during direct laryngoscopy [48, 49] without using Magill forceps.

Observational studies using MIST reported a reduction in the need of MV in 25–28 weeks' gestation babies with a similar trend at 29–32 weeks' gestation.

Although these minimally invasive modes of administering surfactant are promising, their feasibility needs to be better established, especially in the periviable period.

2.6. Early use of caffeine

The early use of caffeine, which has been used for many years to treat apnea of prematurity, seems to be a promising approach. Early treatment (2 vs. 12 h of life) is associated with improved blood pressure and superior vena cava flow without any differences in need for intubation or vasopressors in a small cohort of preterm infants [52].

Moreover, when caffeine is administered early in the DR, it has shown to be effective in increasing spontaneous breathing. Moreover, Dekker et al have found that caffeine enhances the GA-related increase in minute ventilation, and that the stimulatory effect of caffeine on minute ventilation increases with GA [53].

To date, international guidelines do not suggest caffeine administration in the DR, due to lack of extensive studies. However, further evidence is needed to verify its efficacy and benefits when used earlier.

2.7. Practical suggestions:

1. Provide initial alveolar recruitment (using PEEP, short SI, prolonged SI in research setting)
2. Evaluate the presence and efficacy of spontaneous breathing and provide the ventilatory support accordingly:
   - CPAP: **PEEP** = 6 cmH_2O, FiO_2
   - PPV: peak inspiratory pressure (**PIP)** = 25–30 cmH_2O **PEEP** 6 cmH_2O **RR** 40–60 bpm
3. Evaluate response to mask ventilation and titrate support accordingly
   - HR (>100 bpm)
   - SpO_2 (consider postnatal range values)
   - If available, use $ETCO_2$ device and RFM to verify gas exchange and exhaled V_T (V_{Te})
4. Consider surfactant administration
5. Assure maintenance of recruitment during transport to NICU (PPV/CPAP delivered with mask or endotracheal tube or prongs)

2.8. Cord clamping

The current neonatal resuscitation guidelines recommend in term infants delayed cord clamping (DCC) for at least 30 s, although the optimal timing is poorly studied. DCC as opposed to early cord clamping is associated with increased birthweights, hemoglobin levels at 24–48 h, iron stores at 3–6 months [54] and reduced hospital mortality [55]. However, there are some areas of concern surrounding DCC.

Babies undergoing DCC seem to be more likely to need phototherapy for jaundice. It is hypothesized that DCC babies will have a greater incidence of hyperbilirubinemia due to increased iron stores. Pending further evidence, this is an important aspect to consider in settings where kernicterus is common.

Regarding the influence of DCC on respiratory mechanics, there is lack of evidence. A Cochrane review found that babies receiving DCC babies are no more at risk than ICC infants of developing RDS [56], despite limited numbers of studies included and the small size population.

When a baby requires resuscitation or shows clinical conditions, which suggest medical interventions, DCC is not recommended. Thus, under specific circumstances (severe respiratory failure, asphyxia, etc.) an alternative maneuver called "*cord milking*" has been proposed. It consists of stripping the umbilical cord approximately 20–40 cm once or several times (2–4) from the placental end toward the proximal site of the cord. It can be performed in few seconds either while the cord is still attached to the placenta or not.

Whether cord milking is a valid alternative to cord clamping is still under investigation. However, in a population of term infants, early cord clamping with cord milking has shown to increase hemoglobin concentration and iron stores at 6 months of age [57]. The same procedure in late preterm infants is associated with improved iron stores at 6 weeks but also increases the risk of jaundice needing phototherapy [58].

There is paucity of evidence regarding the effects of cord milking on neurodevelopmental outcomes.

2.9. Monitoring during neonatal transition

Although the use of multiple devices monitoring resuscitation (pulse oximetry, ECG, respiratory function monitor-RFM, end-tidal CO_2, NIRS) is still challenging in the DR, there is an increasing interest in monitoring physiologic changes during neonatal transition [59–62].

When preterm infants need respiratory assistance in the delivery room, RFM is desirable to deliver adequate and gentle resuscitation maneuvers and to identify potential pitfalls during mask ventilation [63]. However, establishing this approach may be technically challenging.

Despite all the efforts to optimize resuscitation by the neonatologists, there are several situations in which the efficacy of PPV or CPAP mask ventilation is compromised.

Mask leaks, airways obstructions (e.g., laryngeal closure [64]), interruptions of ventilation due to drying or hat placing are just some examples of how the ventilation can lose efficacy and be suboptimal [65] to deliver a safe and appropriate Vt.

Moreover, the majority of VLBW infants often show a respiratory effort, which is difficult to evaluate, making the decision to start PPV or use CPAP only particularly tricky. Especially in these babies, delivering the adequate Vt is fundamental, because of the high risk of damaging the lung with volutrauma. Measuring the Vt, in fact, is not currently possible without specific devices.

The RFM (**Figure 4**) can integrate and show in real-time information about pulse oximetry and the main respiratory data, reflecting the efficacy of the resuscitation maneuvers. Particularly, a pneumotachometer connecting the resuscitator device and the patient interface provides data of delivered pressures and flows [66, 67] (**Figure 5**). Integration of the flow signal offers data on inspiratory and expiratory tidal volumes (Vti and V_{Te}). This information helps the neonatologist in changing the PIP level to achieve adequate ventilation (**Figure 2**). Moreover, real-time observation of the flow signal is useful to detect face mask leaks or obstructions, which significantly influence a successful mask ventilation. In addition, the flow signal can help in verifying the efficacy of endotracheal intubation.

Upon informed parental consent, RFM can also be used in debriefing sessions of the resuscitation team or for educational purposes, since it is able to video-record the DR stabilization process.

However, RFM does not provide information about the success of lung aeration.

Carbon dioxide (CO_2) levels are good indicators of efficacy in gas exchange [68], and for this reason, colourimetric CO_2 detector is currently used to detect the correct placement of the endotracheal tube [69–71].

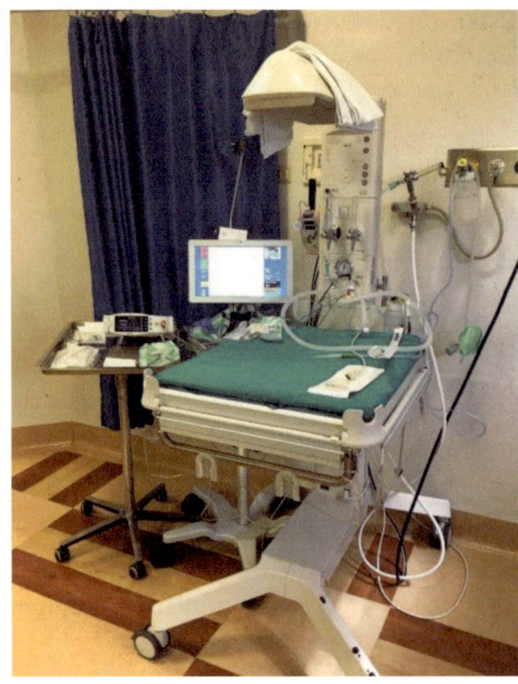

Figure 4. Resuscitation setting with RFM.

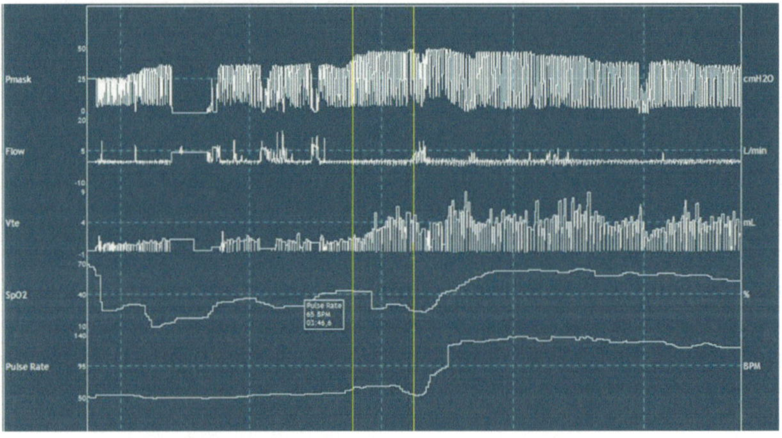

Figure 5. The picture describes the signals recorded by an RFM during stabilization of a preterm infant in the DR. The signal of pressures delivered during mask PPV is indicated as Pmask, expired tidal Volume calculation (V_{Te}), flow signal, pulse rate, and oxygen saturation (SpO_2) are recorded concurrently. Pulse rate and SpO_2 raise in this example is clearly related to raise in peak pressures during mask PPV with a following increase in V_{Te}.

To date, several observational studies have reported the value of using exhaled CO_2 measurement to assess lung aeration and guide respiratory support in the DR [59, 68].

Even if it is a new technique, which must be further investigated to be standardized as a routine practice in the DR, $ETCO_2$ monitoring has been recently shown to be a promising measurement to evaluate the degree of lung aeration and the onset of gas exchange. Moreover, it has been successfully used to monitor SI maneuver during resuscitation [38].

While peripheral oxygen saturation is easily monitored by pulse oximetry and is routine in the DR, Near-infrared spectroscopy (NIRS) allows noninvasive continuous real-time measurement of the regional tissue oxygen saturation. Hence, using NIRS has the potential to monitor cerebral oxygen delivery [72]. Having this information during resuscitation of preterm babies with RDS, could optimize the use of oxygen in the DR and reduce its potential damages.

All the techniques described are potentially intriguing, but further evidence is needed to apply them into routine clinical practice in the DR.

3. Summary

Preterm infants at birth have to face with several limitations, which are inversely proportional to their gestational age. Moreover, prenatal factors play a crucial role in the prognosis and can guide the clinicians in the decision-making process, as early as in the DR.

Antenatal steroids prophylaxis, maternal complications (e.g., diabetes or gestosis) or intrauterine growth restriction may influence surfactant synthesis and storage, mode of delivery and use of general anesthesia may interfere in fetal-neonatal transition and therefore must be considered when the baby is about to be delivered and when resuscitation starts. If RDS signs are already present at birth, several interventions can be adopted to optimize cardio-respiratory management, to improve gas exchange and therefore oxygenation.

An appropriate management from birth, in fact, should lead to the achievement of an early FRC and the following steps should aim at maintaining an adequate lung volume facilitating a more stable systemic and cerebral hemodynamics.

Literature underlines the importance of a tailored respiratory management of preterm infants from birth and during the whole NICU stay to reduce mortality rate and occurrence of severe respiratory (e.g., BPD) and neurological sequelae (e.g., intraventricular hemorrage and periventricular leukomalacia).

Author details

Gianluca Lista[1], Georg M. Schmölzer[2,3]* and Ilia Bresesti[1]

*Address all correspondence to: georg.schmoelzer@me.com

1 Division of Neonatology, "V.Buzzi Children's Hospital", ASST-FBF-Sacco, Milan, Italy

2 Centre for the Studies of Asphyxia and Resuscitation, Royal Alexandra Hospital, Edmonton, Canada

3 Division of Neonatology, Department of Pediatrics, University of Alberta, Edmonton, Canada

References

[1] Hooper SB, Te Pas AB, Kitchen MJ. Respiratory transition in the newborn: A three-phase process. Archives of Disease in Childhood. Fetal and Neonatal Edition. 2016;**101**:F266-F271

[2] Costeloe K, Hennessy E, Gibson AT, Marlow N, Wilkinson AR. The EPICure study: Outcomes to discharge from hospital for infants born at the threshold of viability. Pediatrics. 2000;**106**:659-671

[3] Laptook AR, Salhab W, Bhaskar B. Admission temperature of low birth weight infants: Predictors and associated morbidities. Pediatrics. 2007;**119**:e643-e649

[4] Silverman WA, Fertig JW, Berger AP. The influence of the thermal environment upon the survival of newly born premature infants. Pediatrics. 1958;**22**:876-886

[5] Wyllie J, Perlman JM, Kattwinkel J, Wyckoff MH, Aziz K, Guinsburg R, Kim HS, Liley HG, Mildenhall L, Simon WM, Szyld E, Tamura M, Velaphi S. Part 7: Neonatal resuscitation: 2015 International Consensus on Cardiopulmonary Resuscitation and Emergency Cardiovascular Care Science with Treatment Recommendations. Resuscitation. 2015;**95**: e169-e201

[6] Trevisanuto D, Doglioni N, Cavallin F, Parotto M, Micaglio M, Zanardo V. Heat loss prevention in very preterm infants in delivery rooms: a prospective, randomized, controlled trial of polyethylene caps. The Journal of Pediatrics. 2010;**156**:914-917, 917.e911

[7] McCall EM, Alderdice F, Halliday HL, Jenkins JG, Vohra S. Interventions to prevent hypothermia at birth in preterm and/or low birthweight infants. Cochrane Database of Systematic Reviews. 2010 Mar 17;(3):CD004210

[8] Sweet DG, Carnielli V, Greisen G, Hallman M, Ozek E, Plavka R, Saugstad OD, Simeoni U, Speer CP, Vento M, Visser GH, Halliday HL. European Consensus Guidelines on the Management of Respiratory Distress Syndrome - 2016 Update Neonatology. Basel, Switzerland: S. Karger AG; 2017. pp. 107-125

[9] Jobe AH. Lung maturation: The survival miracle of very low birth weight infants. Pediatrics and Neonatology. 2010;**51**:7-13

[10] Lista G, Maturana A, Moya FR. Achieving and maintaining lung volume in the preterm infant: From the first breath to the NICU. European Journal of Pediatrics. 2017

[11] Morley CJ, Davis PG, Doyle LW, Brion LP, Hascoet JM, Carlin JB. Nasal CPAP or intubation at birth for very preterm infants. The New England Journal of Medicine. 2008; **358**:700-708

[12] Schmölzer GM, Kumar M, Pichler G, Aziz K, O'Reilly M, Cheung PY. Non-invasive versus invasive respiratory support in preterm infants at birth: Systematic review and meta-analysis. BMJ. 2013;**347**:f5980

[13] Dunn MS, Kaempf J, de Klerk A, de Klerk R, Reilly M, Howard D, Ferrelli K, O'Conor J, Soll RF. Randomized trial comparing 3 approaches to the initial respiratory management of preterm neonates. Pediatrics. 2011;**128**:e1069-e1076

[14] Wyllie J, Bruinenberg J, Roehr CC, Rudiger M, Trevisanuto D, Urlesberger B. European Resuscitation Council Guidelines for Resuscitation 2015: Section 7. Resuscitation and support of transition of babies at birth. Resuscitation. 2015;**95**:249-263

[15] Tingay DG, Bhatia R, Schmölzer GM, Wallace MJ, Zahra VA, Davis PG. Effect of sustained inflation vs. stepwise PEEP strategy at birth on gas exchange and lung mechanics in preterm lambs. Pediatric Research. 2014;**75**:288-294

[16] Mehler K, Grimme J, Abele J, Huenseler C, Roth B, Kribs A. Outcome of extremely low gestational age newborns after introduction of a revised protocol to assist preterm infants in their transition to extrauterine life. Acta Paediatrica. 2012;**101**:1232-1239

[17] Peterson J, Johnson N, Deakins K, Wilson-Costello D, Jelovsek JE, Chatburn R. Accuracy of the 7-8-9 Rule for endotracheal tube placement in the neonate. Journal of Perinatology. 2006;**26**:333-336

[18] Yam CH, Dawson JA, Schmölzer GM, Morley CJ, Davis PG. Heart rate changes during resuscitation of newly born infants <30 weeks gestation: An observational study. Archives of Disease in Childhood. Fetal and Neonatal Edition. 2011;**96**:F102-F107

[19] Perlman JM, Wyllie J, Kattwinkel J, Atkins DL, Chameides L, Goldsmith JP, Guinsburg R, Hazinski MF, Morley C, Richmond S, Simon WM, Singhal N, Szyld E, Tamura M, Velaphi S. Part 11: Neonatal resuscitation: 2010 International Consensus on Cardiopulmonary Resuscitation and Emergency Cardiovascular Care Science With Treatment Recommendations. Circulation. 2010;**122**:S516-S538

[20] Chitkara R, Rajani AK, Oehlert JW, Lee HC, Epi MS, Halamek LP. The accuracy of human senses in the detection of neonatal heart rate during standardized simulated resuscitation: Implications for delivery of care, training and technology design. Resuscitation. 2013; **84**:369-372

[21] Mizumoto H, Tomotaki S, Shibata H, Ueda K, Akashi R, Uchio H, Hata D. Electrocardiogram shows reliable heart rates much earlier than pulse oximetry during neonatal resuscitation. Pediatrics International. 2012;**54**:205-207

[22] Voogdt KG, Morrison AC, Wood FE, van Elburg RM, Wyllie JP. A randomised, simulated study assessing auscultation of heart rate at birth. Resuscitation. 2010;**81**:1000-1003

[23] Kamlin CO, O'Donnell CP, Everest NJ, Davis PG, Morley CJ. Accuracy of clinical assessment of infant heart rate in the delivery room. Resuscitation. 2006;**71**:319-321

[24] Kamlin CO, Dawson JA, O'Donnell CP, Morley CJ, Donath SM, Sekhon J, Davis PG. Accuracy of pulse oximetry measurement of heart rate of newborn infants in the delivery room. The Journal of Pediatrics. 2008;**152**:756-760

[25] Saugstad OD, Ramji S, Soll RF, Vento M. Resuscitation of newborn infants with 21% or 100% oxygen: an updated systematic review and meta-analysis. Neonatology. 2008; **94**:176-182

[26] Wang CL, Anderson C, Leone TA, Rich W, Govindaswami B, Finer NN. Resuscitation of preterm neonates by using room air or 100% oxygen. Pediatrics. 2008;**121**:1083-1089

[27] McCall KE, Davis PG, Owen LS, Tingay DG. Sustained lung inflation at birth: What do we know, and what do we need to know? Archives of Disease in Childhood. Fetal and Neonatal Edition. 2016;**101**:F175-F180

[28] te Pas AB, Siew M, Wallace MJ, Kitchen MJ, Fouras A, Lewis RA, Yagi N, Uesugi K, Donath S, Davis PG, Morley CJ, Hooper SB. Establishing functional residual capacity at birth: The effect of sustained inflation and positive end-expiratory pressure in a preterm rabbit model. Pediatric Research. 2009;**65**:537-541

[29] Fuchs H, Lindner W, Buschko A, Trischberger T, Schmid M, Hummler HD. Cerebral oxygenation in very low birth weight infants supported with sustained lung inflations after birth. Pediatric Research. 2011;**70**:176-180

[30] Vyas H, Milner AD, Hopkin IE, Boon AW. Physiologic responses to prolonged and slow-rise inflation in the resuscitation of the asphyxiated newborn infant. The Journal of Pediatrics. 1981;**99**:635-639

[31] Lista G, Boni L, Scopesi F, Mosca F, Trevisanuto D, Messner H, Vento G, Magaldi R, Del Vecchio A, Agosti M, Gizzi C, Sandri F, Biban P, Bellettato M, Gazzolo D, Boldrini A, Dani C. Sustained lung inflation at birth for preterm infants: A randomized clinical trial. Pediatrics. 2015;**135**:e457-e464

[32] van Vonderen JJ, Hooper SB, Hummler HD, Lopriore E, te Pas AB. Effects of a sustained inflation in preterm infants at birth. The Journal of Pediatrics. 2014;**165** 903-908.e901

[33] Sobotka KS, Hooper SB, Allison BJ, Te Pas AB, Davis PG, Morley CJ, Moss TJ. An initial sustained inflation improves the respiratory and cardiovascular transition at birth in preterm lambs. Pediatric Research. 2011;**70**:56-60

[34] Harding R, Bocking AD, Sigger JN. Influence of upper respiratory tract on liquid flow to and from fetal lungs. Journal of Applied Physiology. (1985) 1986;**61**:68-74

[35] Lista G, Cavigioli F, La Verde PA, Castoldi F, Bresesti I, Morley CJ. Effects of breathing and apnoea during sustained inflations in resuscitation of preterm infants. Neonatology. 2017;**111**:360-366

[36] Lindner W, Vossbeck S, Hummler H, Pohlandt F. Delivery room management of extremely low birth weight infants: Spontaneous breathing or intubation? Pediatrics. 1999;**103**:961-967

[37] te Pas AB, Walther FJ. A randomized, controlled trial of delivery-room respiratory management in very preterm infants. Pediatrics. 2007;**120**:322-329

[38] Ngan AY, Cheung PY, Hudson-Mason A, O'Reilly M, van Os S, Kumar M, Aziz K, Schmölzer GM. Using exhaled CO2 to guide initial respiratory support at birth: A randomised controlled trial. Archives of Disease in Childhood. Fetal and Neonatal Edition. 2017;**102**:F525-f531

[39] Keszler M. Sustained inflation during neonatal resuscitation. Current Opinion in Pediatrics. 2015;**27**:145-151

[40] Wyckoff MH, Aziz K, Escobedo MB, Kapadia VS, Kattwinkel J, Perlman JM, Simon WM, Weiner GM, Zaichkin JG. Part 13: Neonatal Resuscitation: 2015 American Heart Association Guidelines Update for Cardiopulmonary Resuscitation and Emergency Cardiovascular Care. Circulation. 2015;**132**:S543-S560

[41] Rojas-Reyes MX, Morley CJ, Soll R. Prophylactic versus selective use of surfactant in preventing morbidity and mortality in preterm infants. Cochrane Database of Systematic Reviews. 2012 Mar 14;(3):CD000510

[42] Subramaniam P, Ho JJ, Davis PG. Prophylactic nasal continuous positive airway pressure for preventing morbidity and mortality in very preterm infants. Cochrane Database of Systematic Reviews 2016 Jun 14;(6):CD001243

[43] Fischer HS, Buhrer C. Avoiding endotracheal ventilation to prevent bronchopulmonary dysplasia: A meta-analysis. Pediatrics. 2013;**132**:e1351-e1360

[44] Finer NN, Carlo WA, Duara S, Fanaroff AA, Donovan EF, Wright LL, Kandefer S, Poole WK, Network NIoCHaHDNR. Delivery room continuous positive airway pressure/positive end-expiratory pressure in extremely low birth weight infants: A feasibility trial. Pediatrics. 2004;**114**:651-657

[45] Bahadue FL, Soll R. Early versus delayed selective surfactant treatment for neonatal respiratory distress syndrome. Cochrane Database of Systematic Reviews. 2012;**11**:CD001456

[46] Walsh MC, Morris BH, Wrage LA, Vohr BR, Poole WK, Tyson JE, Wright LL, Ehrenkranz RA, Stoll BJ, Fanaroff AA. Extremely low birthweight neonates with protracted ventilation: Mortality and 18-month neurodevelopmental outcomes. The Journal of Pediatrics. 2005;**146**:798-804

[47] Gopel W, Kribs A, Ziegler A, Laux R, Hoehn T, Wieg C, Siegel J, Avenarius S, von der Wense A, Vochem M, Groneck P, Weller U, Moller J, Hartel C, Haller S, Roth B, Herting E. Avoidance of mechanical ventilation by surfactant treatment of spontaneously breathing preterm infants (AMV): An open-label, randomised, controlled trial. Lancet. 2011;**378**:1627-1634

[48] Dargaville PA, Aiyappan A, De Paoli AG, Kuschel CA, Kamlin CO, Carlin JB, Davis PG. Minimally-invasive surfactant therapy in preterm infants on continuous positive airway pressure. Archives of Disease in Childhood. Fetal and Neonatal Edition. 2013;**98**:F122-F126

[49] Dargaville PA, Aiyappan A, Cornelius A, Williams C, De Paoli AG. Preliminary evaluation of a new technique of minimally invasive surfactant therapy. Archives of Disease in Childhood. Fetal and Neonatal Edition. 2011;**96**:F243-F248

[50] Kribs A, Pillekamp F, Hunseler C, Vierzig A, Roth B. Early administration of surfactant in spontaneous breathing with nCPAP: feasibility and outcome in extremely premature infants (postmenstrual age </=27 weeks). Paediatric Anaesthesia. 2007;**17**:364-369

[51] Kribs A, Vierzig A, Hunseler C, Eifinger F, Welzing L, Stutzer H, Roth B. Early surfactant in spontaneously breathing with nCPAP in ELBW infants–A single centre four year experience. Acta Paediatrica. 2008;**97**:293-298

[52] Katheria AC, Sauberan JB, Akotia D, Rich W, Durham J, Finer NN. A pilot randomized controlled trial of early versus routine caffeine in extremely premature infants. American Journal of Perinatology. 2015;**32**:879-886

[53] Dekker J, Hooper SB, van Vonderen JJ, Witlox RSGM, Lopriore E, Te Pas AB. Caffeine to improve breathing effort of preterm infants at birth: A randomized controlled trial. Pediatric Research. 2017

[54] McDonald SJ, Middleton P, Dowswell T, Morris PS. Effect of timing of umbilical cord clamping of term infants on maternal and neonatal outcomes. Evidence-Based Child Health. 2014;**9**:303-397

[55] Fogarty M, Osborn DA, Askie L, Seidler AL, Hunter K, Lui K, Simes J, Tarnow-Mordi W. Delayed versus early umbilical cord clamping for preterm infants: A systematic review and meta-analysis. American Journal of Obstetrics and Gynecology. 2017

[56] Rabe H, Diaz-Rossello JL, Duley L, Dowswell T. Effect of timing of umbilical cord clamping and other strategies to influence placental transfusion at preterm birth on maternal and infant outcomes. Cochrane Database of Systematic Reviews. 2012 Aug 15;(8):CD003248

[57] Bora R, Akhtar SS, Venkatasubramaniam A, Wolfson J, Rao R. Effect of 40-cm segment umbilical cord milking on hemoglobin and serum ferritin at 6 months of age in full-term infants of anemic and non-anemic mothers. Journal of Perinatology. 2015;**35**:832-836

[58] Kumar B, Upadhyay A, Gothwal S, Jaiswal V, Joshi P, Dubey K. Umbilical cord milking and hematological parameters in moderate to late preterm neonates: A randomized controlled trial. Indian Pediatrics. 2015;**52**:753-757

[59] van Os S, Cheung PY, Pichler G, Aziz K, O'Reilly M, Schmölzer GM. Exhaled carbon dioxide can be used to guide respiratory support in the delivery room. Acta Paediatrica. 2014;**103**:796-806

[60] Mian QN, Pichler G, Binder C, O'Reilly M, Aziz K, Urlesberger B, Cheung PY, Schmölzer GM. Tidal volumes in spontaneously breathing preterm infants supported with continuous positive airway pressure. The Journal of Pediatrics. 2014;**165**:702-706.e701

[61] Pichler G, Cheung PY, Binder C, O'Reilly M, Schwaberger B, Aziz K, Urlesberger B, Schmölzer GM. Time course study of blood pressure in term and preterm infants immediately after birth. PLoS One. 2014;**9**:e114504

[62] Baik N, Urlesberger B, Schwaberger B, Schmölzer GM, Mileder L, Avian A, Pichler G. Reference ranges for cerebral tissue oxygen saturation index in term neonates during immediate neonatal transition after birth. Neonatology. 2015;**108**:283-286

[63] Lista G, Schmölzer G, Colm OD. Improving assessment during noninvasive ventilation in the delivery room. NeoReviews. 2012;**13**:e364-e371

[64] Crawshaw JR, Kitchen MJ, Binder-Heschl C, Thio M, Wallace MJ, Kerr LT, Roehr CC, Lee KL, Buckley GA, Davis PG, Flemmer A, Te Pas AB, Hooper SB. Laryngeal closure impedes non-invasive ventilation at birth. Archives of Disease in Childhood. Fetal and Neonatal Edition. 2017 Oct 20. pii: fetalneonatal-2017-312681. DOI: 10.1136/archdischild-2017-312681

[65] Schmölzer GM, Dawson JA, Kamlin CO, O'Donnell CP, Morley CJ, Davis PG. Airway obstruction and gas leak during mask ventilation of preterm infants in the delivery room. Archives of Disease in Childhood. Fetal and Neonatal Edition. 2011;**96**:F254-F257

[66] Schmölzer GM, Morley CJ, Wong C, Dawson JA, Kamlin CO, Donath SM, Hooper SB, Davis PG. Respiratory function monitor guidance of mask ventilation in the delivery room: A feasibility study. The Journal of Pediatrics. 2012;**160**:377-381.e372

[67] Verbeek C, van Zanten HA, van Vonderen JJ, Kitchen MJ, Hooper SB, Te Pas AB. Accuracy of currently available neonatal respiratory function monitors for neonatal resuscitation. European Journal of Pediatrics. 2016;**175**:1065-1070

[68] Hooper SB, Fouras A, Siew ML, Wallace MJ, Kitchen MJ, te Pas AB, Klingenberg C, Lewis RA, Davis PG, Morley CJ, Schmölzer GM. Expired CO_2 levels indicate degree of lung aeration at birth. PLoS One. 2013;**8**:e70895

[69] Leone TA, Lange A, Rich W, Finer NN. Disposable colorimetric carbon dioxide detector use as an indicator of a patent airway during noninvasive mask ventilation. Pediatrics. 2006;**118**:e202-e204

[70] Schmölzer GM, O'Reilly M, Davis PG, Cheung PY, Roehr CC. Confirmation of correct tracheal tube placement in newborn infants. Resuscitation. 2013;**84**:731-737

[71] Schmölzer GM, Roehr CC. Techniques to ascertain correct endotracheal tube placement in neonates. Cochrane Database of Systematic Reviews. 2014 Sep 13;(9):CD010221

[72] Pichler G, Cheung PY, Aziz K, Urlesberger B, Schmölzer GM. How to monitor the brain during immediate neonatal transition and resuscitation? A systematic qualitative review of the literature. Neonatology. 2014;**105**:205-210